PATIENTS
PROFIT$
&
POWER

*A Documented Commentary On
The State of Health Care Industry*

Harold Stearley, RN

©1996 Harold Stearley, RN

This book is protected by copyright. No part of this book may be reproduced in any form or by any means, including photocopying or utilized by any information storage or retrieval system without written permission from copyright owner and publisher.

The views exposed within this book are exclusively those of the author and do not necessarily reflect the views and opinions of the publisher.

Reprint permission granted from *Columbia Daily Tribune*, *St. Louis Post-Dispatch* and *Columbia Missourian*.

Library of Congress Catalog Card Number: 96-68738

ISBN: 1-888315-01-6

Printed in the United States of America

Cover Design: Pamela Carrasco

Published by
Power Publications
56 McArthur Avenue
Staten Island, New York 10312
1-800-331-6534

987654321

Table of Contents

Introduction		i
Chapter 1	Express Yourself - At Your Own Risk	1
Chapter 2	Healthcare Criminals	11
Chapter 3	Healthcare Reform	15
Chapter 4	Today's Shamans	25
Chapter 5	After The March	27
Chapter 6	Therapeutic Misadventure	33
Chapter 7	Missouri Health Care - Let The Citizen Decide	37
Chapter 8	Patient - Focused Care	41
Chapter 9	Transplantation Can't Immortalize Heroes	49
Chapter 10	The NLRB Versus Healthcare & Retirement Corporation	53
Chapter 11	The Rise and Fall of the Nursing Union	57
Chapter 12	Strike Back!	63
Chapter 13	Seeding, Misleading, Switching, and Stealing:	73
Chapter 14	Home Health and Medicare Another Fox in the Chicken Coop	77
Chapter 15	COMPARED TO WHAT?	81
Chapter 16	Has the Health Care Industry Crash Landed?	85
Chapter 17	Physicians' Image Needs Healing	89
Chapter 18	Tobacco, Healthcare, and Politics	93
Chapter 19	Defensive Nursing	97
Chapter 20	Professional Jealousy - The No Win Factor	105
Chapter 21	Restructuring and the ANA - Who's Side Are They On?	111
Chapter 22	True Lies, True Risks	121
Chapter 23	Battered But Not Beaten - The Politics of Victimization	125
Chapter 24	Medicare Reform - You Bet Your Life	131
Chapter 25	Terminal Chaos	135
Bibliography		139

Introduction

Professional Post Holes

I have borne the brunt of some criticism over the years for growing up in small town U.S.A. After all, how could a country boy like myself know anything of worldly issues? How could I have any knowledge or insight into global perspectives? How could I possibly understand anything about the complex issues surrounding healthcare or have the nerve to write about it? Well, fortunately life doesn't occur in a vacuum, and at risk of sounding all too cliché, I must say I've been around a little.

There are times when I'm more than proud of my simple country lifestyle, and it provides me with more insight than anyone could obtain from the so-called "modern world" filled with "double speak" and "techno-babble."

Not long ago a battle began in my "neck of the woods" regarding a local developer's idea to drop a subdivision right in the middle of small rural community. This just happened to be the small enclave where I live. My neighbors, and myself, all own anywhere from one-half acre to forty acres - a nice "spread out" group of quaint country homes.

It's not uncommon to look out your back door an see several deer wondering through the woods, or coming down to a pond for a drink. It's not uncommon to hear the coyotes howling at the moon, or owls hooting in the middle of the night. It's not uncommon to wake up one morning and discover you have a whole den of red foxes in the brush pile just thirty feet from your front door. Canadian geese, wood ducks, great blue herons, six different species of woodpeckers, sparrow hawks, red-tailed hawks, and even wild turkey abound. Every type of critter imaginable - raccoons, muskrats, beaver, opossum, red and gray squirrels - well you get the idea. It's quiet, it's serene, it's beautiful!

In comes Mr. Money-Hungry Developer and he wants to drop 240 low-income homes (a nice way of saying a glorified trailer-park) right in the middle of this picture of serenity. You can say good-by to the piece and quiet, to the wildlife, and even to the property values.

The, not so sophisticated, country people of my community unified and offered more resistance at the County Planning and Zoning Commission meetings than any nurses in my part of the country have offered against restructuring. The battle lasted a full year with half a dozen meetings discussing the proposed density, the potential for pollution, the quality of the homes, the conditions of roads, and the access of utilities.

In the end, the developer won his subdivision, but it had been whittled down to only 130 homes - all have to have a minimum of half acre sized lots. Not a total victory, but the new neighborhood will retain some of its country atmosphere.

There will be some new liability concerns for those of us accustomed to not having to worry about groups of new small children wondering onto our property and being injured or drowning in a pond or lake (in nursing we have new liability issues related to how restructuring has left us with too few RNs to take care of patients properly). So considerable time, attention, and expense is being expended in the construction of new fences. I'm constructing my own, even as I write this introduction.

So what does all of this have to do with nursing or healthcare in general? Well, this simple country labor of constructing a fence holds some great parallels to determining the directions our profession might take. Nursing professionals could stand to learn a lot from the comparison.

Foundation. Every structure ever constructed must be built on a strong foundation. The same is true of professions, and nursing must strengthen its own foundation if it wishes to survive and support its advancement.

Nursing itself is the foundation for the entire patient care delivery system in this country. The backbone, if you will, upon which all patient care is supported. Sure the physicians are in charge of diagnosing and prescribing, but it's the nurses who continually assess and direct the physicians as to which patient care interventions need to be ordered. It is also the nurses who then perform those interventions.

With a barbed wire fence, the posts serve as the framework for maintaining the entire structure. Especially the corner posts. In fact, the anchored metal posts which compose the majority of the line are merely there to hold up the wire. It's the corner posts which truly provide the strength to bear the weight and tension of the wire. If the corner posts are not placed appropriately the entire construction will twist and collapse under its own weight.

Nursing's models of practice are the corner posts of our scope of practice. Determining which model we practice under ultimately determines the quality of the services we will be able to provide. Thus, total patient care models employing large numbers of RNs promote optimum patient outcome, while Patient-Focused Care models using large numbers of unlicensed, minimally trained assistants result in massive increases in patient morbidity and mortality. Under the current wave of brutal cost-saving initiatives, the foundation of health care delivery is twisting and on the verge of collapse.

When I had to construct my fence, I wanted to be sure it was I who was determining the boundaries of my property. I did not want to sacrifice one inch to that greedy land developer. I hired my own professional surveyors, and had them painstakingly mark off my property line.

With our profession, it should be the staff nurses, the professionals who provide bedside care on a daily basis, who determine our professional boundaries. We should not let any Board of Nursing, any other healthcare professionals, any legislators, any hospital administrators, or any national association dictate to us how we can practice nor what the limits of our practice should be. We are the ones who know how to care for our patients, and we should not give up 1 centimeter of our practice to another group of health care workers - especially unlicensed assistive personnel.

Once my boundaries were delineated, I had to clear the obstacles which prevented me from building my fence. It took four passes with my brush-cutter and chain saw to eliminate the underbrush, the fallen logs, and the sturdy trees which blocked the path of my construction.

Nurses too must eliminate the obstacles which are blocking their practice. They must channel their support to organizations which truly support nurses' mission of the highest quality patient care. Has the ANA lived up to this obligation? In a future chapter we will examine their tacit support for the replacement of RNs with UAP.

Nurses must not allow themselves to be intimidated by administrators who threaten and coerce. Nurses must take their battles for safe patient care to their legislators. Nurses must convince the public that their skills for treating them can not be replaced by unlicensed personnel. Nurses must sharpen their chain saws and brush cutters and clear their path of all who threaten to de-license or dismantle their practice. Dig in for a long battle for it may take more than four passes with heavy equipment to clear our paths.

The labor was tedious in preparing my fence line. I measured the total length which needed to be spanned with the heavy gauge, four-pointed wire. I placed markers for each post - no greater than eight feet apart to support the load. I drove each anchored metal "T-post" (named for their shape) exactly 18 inches into the ground to attain both maximum support and the proper height to hold the wire appropriately. And finally I came to the corner posts.

The corner posts are milled pine logs. They are eight inches in diameter and eight feet long. They are pressure treated with a creosote product to prevent them from rotting in the elements. This treatment increases their weight to approximately 200 pounds each. These are the primary supports for the entire fence structure. These are our models of practice which support the nurses, which in turn support the entire healthcare delivery system. Placed the wrong way the system collapses upon itself. The wrong nursing care model and your patient's health collapses right in front of you.

The placement of these corner posts is crucial. Crucial, you ask? Why so important? Well, to set the post appropriately a hole must be dug. It is dug three feet deep, one foot in diameter, and it must be straight down forming a 90 degree angle with the ground. It must be in right spot - for you see, once dug, you can't move a post hole. Sounds simplistic doesn't it, but remember the corner posts will support the entire structure.

Once you drag your 200 pound post through the cleared pathway, you have cut, you must place it in the hole perfectly perpendicular to the ground. You add 120 pounds of concrete mix, and fill the remaining opening with the dirt you had extracted. But don't think you're done yet.

The corner posts are placed in a triangular formation - three to each corner. They are further supported by notching them with your chain saw, inserting a cross timber, and "X wiring" this configuration with number 9 gauge galvanized steel wire. This wiring places an inward tension on the posts which is balanced by the outward pressure from the cross beam between them. The foundation, once completed, is as solid as a rock.

Why so much trouble for these corner posts? You don't just hang the barbed wire as it will sag under its own heavy weight. The wire is stretched tight per a specially designed tool, and while stretched you apply the metal clamps which hold the wire to each post for the length of the entire fence. When this wire is stretched, it is no longer just the weight which is supported by the posts - you now have an additional force of tension. The direction of the tension is inward - from corner post to corner post, and as the slack is pulled from the wire these foundation posts must balance this tension. If they do not hold, the posts buckle, the wire twists, and the force topples the entire line. I've seen the metal T posts ripped from the ground by the recoiling force of stretched barbed wire snapping back into its original coil.

So how on earth did we end up talking about fences? Well, as our national nursing leaders determine the models under which we practice nursing, remember they are digging our professional post holes. Also remember, once dug, these holes cannot be moved. These holes provide the support for our foundation of corner posts. These corner posts carry the load, and delineate the boundaries for our entire practice. And, its our practice, the practice of nursing, which is the foundation of all health care delivery in this country.

If our professional foundation is improperly designed, the profession itself will twist, buckle, and collapse - and if we go, so do our patients. We cannot move our professional post-holes, so to place them in the wrong spot merely creates more work for us as we must then rebuild our foundations, and redefine our practice boundaries. Nursing would be a much stronger profession if we weren't always having to start over with the latest management concocted delivery scheme designed to sacrifice patients in the name of profit.

As nurses we provide the backbone of the entire healthcare industry. Our models of practice determine the quality of the care we are going to be able to provide. As the practitioners of bedside care, nurses must determine the direction of their profession. We must determine our own models of practice - the ones which align themselves with patient advocacy.

As you read the following chapters, keep in mind that the nursing profession is under siege. We are being attacked on all fronts - nursing and hospital administrators, for-profit corporations, nursing associations, physicians, and nursing academia. Sometimes we even undermine ourselves, and sometimes this occurs when we trust others to make our decisions for us.

Staff nurses have only one interest at heart - caring for people. We should not allow these other special interest groups to dig our professional post-holes. Our role is far too important to trust others to define it. We own our licenses and we own our profession - but only if we decide to take control of it. The challenge is formidable, but then again so is the art of healing.......

Chapter 1

Express Yourself - At Your Own Risk

If you could be "a fly on the wall" in today's hospital you would hear startling stories regarding the treatment of patients - and nurses. Tales of physician malpractice and negligence. Tales of administrative incompetence and abuse. Tales of profit maximizing strategies which put patients at risk, and end professional careers. Then again, maybe these stories have always been around. Only now, in the age of health care reform, public scrutiny of this traditionally closed-door industry is beginning to expose some of these tales of medical horror. In this current political climate nurses have been raising their voices to put patients above profits - but at what personal sacrifice?

Nurses have always been at the forefront, using whatever powers they have to overcome the inadequacies encountered in their institutions of healing. The goal has always been to provide exceptional care - no matter how short the staffing, how poor the equipment, how unsupportive the management, or how abusive the physician. Nurses speak of these challenges and obstacles daily - amongst themselves. Even with the growth of nursing publications, and nursing authors, the over-all numbers of public advocates remains small. Why?

While nurses can attest to the fact they have been quiet too long, there seems to be an inherent fear to speak up -especially publicly. Nursing administrators, and physicians, have been ruling by intimidation for many years, and the threat of losing one's livelihood for expressing an opinion, no matter how strong one's conviction may be, remains a potent threat indeed. In fact, when I joined the ranks of nurse authors, and published a few editorials in our local newspaper, the first opposition I received came from my peers. "You can't say that!" "Why did you write this?" "Who do you think you are?" "Why did you use your real name?" "Just what is your agenda anyway?" I was surprised, and even though I pointed out that they themselves had voiced the same complaints, my peers still replied that it was only appropriate to speak behind closed doors. I was fascinated. The nurses I worked with seemed more than happy to cover-up all of the abuses within their own system. These same bedside advocates were unwilling to go public, were unwilling to attempt to change the system, and basically were scared to death of what would happen to them if they spoke out.

2   Patients Profits & Power

Well the questions from my peers, and superiors, have never stopped coming - and neither has my writing. You see, freedom of expression is guaranteed by the U.S. Constitution, and exercising our civil rights is what makes this country the best in the world. Challenging the norm, the accepted practice, the rut we work in, is what can bring about positive change. My hat is off to Revolution - The Journal of Nurse Empowerment for embracing a philosophy of examination - examination of the problems in our profession, and examination of alternatives and solutions to those problems. Yes, it is difficult to change a situation if you deny its existence. But in my mind it is even worse to cover the problem up, make excuses, or simply run away from it.

I have learned the real power to make changes in medical practice lies with the consumer. If you can educate the consumer, then she/he will demand the changes required to improve the delivery of health care. Nurses couldn't be in a more perfect position to educate patients. We educate them at the bedside daily. We teach patients how to care for themselves. We assist them with asking the physicians to explain their procedures and treatments. Why not take these efforts a step further and educate potential patients before they arrive at the hospital seeking treatment? Why not openly examine the issues, good or bad, and allow the consumer to make a truly informed decision as to what is appropriate health care? Taking a stand, especially a public stand, on any issue is not an easy task, but it is a necessary one for those of us who truly wish to call ourselves patient advocates.

While I strongly urge all nurses to speak out, I'll have to acknowledge there are real dangers encountered when doing so. I would like to relate some strategies I have learned along the way. Personal experience, which can, possibly, smooth out some of the pot holes for those of you who decide to ride this road, and accept the risks of expressing one's opinion.

Not long, several hours to be exact, after my peers responded to my articles I was approached by my superiors. Intimidation was their tactic of choice, and here is how they applied it...

My first editorial to appear concerned the issues surrounding physician performance of unnecessary tests, procedures, and surgeries. The day it appeared, several co-workers asked me to obtain copies for them. I encouraged those asking to obtain their own copies, but I made the mistake of giving out two copies to fellow nurses. A physician noticed them reading the article, noticed the title of the article, and proceeded to walk up to me and remove a copy from my hands without even a word of request. Two lines into the article he blurted, "Who is this guy?" When another nurse explained it was the person he had stolen the paper from, he stormed out of the room. He refused to discuss the article with its author, but returned to the unit, pulled another nurse aside, and began discussing it with her. This discussion occurred approximately ten feet away from me, lasted 3 minutes, or less, and could not be heard by any other staff member.

The following day I received a phone call from my supervisor. She informed me that I was in serious trouble. I was facing possible termination because the manager of the unit in question claimed the article interfered with patient care. Thus, the absurdity began, and would follow me for at least two more years. I was instructed to report to work early for a high level management meeting. Prior to the meeting, I discussed the issue with a co-worker to gain another perspective. This co-worker worked in the same unit where the alleged incident occurred, and thus worked for the manager filing the complaint against me. Unknown to myself, after my discussion with this staff nurse, she approached the accusing manger to express her disbelief of the harassment I was receiving - a big mistake. When I arrived for the meeting I was issued a verbal warning for distributing material on the hospital's premises which was "contrary to the institution's philosophy of the multi-disciplinary team approach to patient care." If this wasn't a major stretch of the imagination in itself, I was informed that by discussing the issue with my co-worker that I had interfered with that particular manager's ability to manage her staff.

I was instructed to never discuss any issue with any other staff member. While these administrators were careful to tip-toe around my right to express my opinion publicly, it was strongly suggested that I keep my ideas to myself. Even though the institution sold the local newspapers in two separate locations, I was instructed that I could not purchase a newspaper and give it to another employee. I was surprised at just how violent their reaction was, especially since the editorial concerned physicians - not nurses. Why were the nursing administrators persecuting me? I thought that we, as nurses, were on the same team.

Several weeks later, I received a document concerning this "verbal warning", a copy of which was placed in my personnel file. The only remarks administration put in writing were, 1) I was accused of contriving the opinion that my job was in jeopardy - no one had called to inform me of this, 2) I had copied the article at my own expense - thus not using any institutional resources which would have been "a conflict of interest" requiring immediate termination, and 3) I was warned not to distribute such materials on work time. They were extremely careful to leave the bulk of the meeting's discussions off the record. This allowed them an element of deniability - to be able to state that no harassment had occurred.

What I had learned from this first round was nursing managers, hospital administrators, and physicians were on the same team - the money-making team, and any perceived threat to their cash flow was to be eliminated. First Amendment Rights, and patient care, were only secondary concerns, and only their opinions were the correct ones. I now understood the physicians exercised a great deal of leverage over nursing administration, and since doctors are the gate-keepers for patient-dollars, the administration offers up what ever sacrifices they desire on a silver platter. Nurses, on the other hand, are regarded as the "B Team", and like children, are "better seen and not heard." In an attempt to restore some perspective, I had pointed out that my editorial could largely be found in the local recycling bins, and did not pose a threat to their patient inventory. However, words are perceived to be very powerful, and I was about to learn just how far administration would go to silence an employee.

At the early stage of this internal commotion I still had a couple of friends in management positions, and what they reported to me was chilling to say the least. In the course of regular management meetings, I was being portrayed as a poor worker. Upper administration was informed that I was lazy, and a "smart a..." This commentary was being propagated by managers who did not even know me, who new nothing of my extensive education, work performance, or any other hard earned accomplishments. This type of closed door, stabbing in the back, communication style is very effective, however, and it turned management, in general, against me. These same managers focused their next attack on my peers.

Suddenly, I had nurses from various departments informing me they were instructed not to associate with me at the risk of destroying their own careers. It was said that I was "poison." This type of character assassination is slanderous, and represents a defamation of character, both of which are illegal, but apparently familiar tactics of this all out extermination program. Obviously, it is unpleasant to report to work each day when your administration is out to harass you, but when your colleagues are afraid to be seen speaking to you it makes for a very uncomfortable working environment.

The next incident occurred three months later when I was informed I was ineligible for a merit raise because of the warning I had received for distributing my editorial. I was reminded about the write-up which inhabited my personnel file. Of course, this action had nothing to do with me expressing my opinions, and after making this statement, my manager did give me a "token" raise - not enough to pay for parking, but enough to prevent me from being able to file a lawsuit. The message was clear, "continue to speak up and we'll continue to make things very difficult for you."

Six months after my original article, a second was published concerning variations in institutional prices for medical procedures. This time I was called in and informed that I would need to attend "mandatory re-education sessions." The last time I had heard such terminology was concerning Mao Tse-tung's re-education program in Communist China. By this time, I had retained an attorney, and was well informed as to what my rights were, and how they were being violated. The words harassment, defamation, slander, grievance, and attorney were dropped to various individuals, and miraculously I attended one "voluntary" meeting with "institutional experts" to discuss the issues raised by the editorial. Even these "medical experts" expressed their confusion as to why this meeting was even occurring. Later I found out that pressure, by the physicians, had been placed on certain managers "to do something" about this "problem."

My next article focused on the lobbying efforts of physicians, drug companies, and insurance organizations to prevent any type of health care reform. One day after this article appeared, I was informed that my position would be eliminated - for budgetary reasons. At first I was simply told "good luck." A month later I was informed that due to my seniority they would find me something, but during my internal interviews one manager informed me that my writing was very controversial and she did not wish to hire a "trouble maker." Another told me that she had been instructed not to hire me by the Director of Nursing, and the third simply stated, "I would have to think long and hard before I ever hired you." I discovered later that persons with less qualifications were hired for two of those three positions. Interestingly enough, during my interviews there were never any questions asked about my education, experience, or certifications. The only questions I was asked regarded my interpersonal relationship skills. I had three job interviews in which the conversation never once focused on the jobs in question, or my ability to perform those jobs!

So just where did I stand? Unfortunately, as my attorney informed me, labor law doesn't always protect employees in the manner in which it should. Filing a grievance would be difficult, simply because it would be hard to prove all of this harassment was occurring. After all, the administration had been careful not to put anything in writing. But then again, I had taken certain precautions myself, and had maintained a journal of all of the events which had transpired. And even if the courts would fail me, there is one thing which hospitals despise even more than vocal nurses, and that is bad publicity. This is one story they did not want to break.

The next step of the harassment was to cut my pay - by an appreciable amount! I suppose it was believed that, during the interim of awaiting a new position, I would simply get fed-up and leave. In fact, I was constantly encouraged to leave. "Oh, you're still here?" "Any luck finding a new job yet, we don't want to stand in your way of moving on." "We wouldn't want you to pass up another opportunity." All the while this "encouragement" was occurring, I had heard, from friends, that it had already been decided to reinstate my position. It was preferred, however, that I not be in it. Ironically, it was the physicians, I worked with closely, who came to my position's defense. No one could figure out a better way to provide nursing coverage for the patients under care from my department. They were unwilling to give up the nursing coverage, not necessarily me in particular, but they required a nurse to assist with their procedures. My position was fully reinstated, six months after its elimination. Again, it is clear just who has the power in the health care arena - the wishes of physicians will over-ride any administrative decisions.

So, as it turned out, I did not have to file a grievance, or a lawsuit. None the less, my attorney was prepared, and remains so to this day. Had I not prepared my articles with some forethought, I would not have had the opportunity to hang on for any type of position. It seems there are certain things employers can do without consequence. Most states have "Employment at Will" statues which allow employers the freedom to terminate you without any cause at all. There are exceptions to this rule, however, and there are techniques which further help to protect your right to free speech. Here are some of the strategies I employed to further protect my rights, and I will illustrate with a few legal briefs to demonstrate just how important it is to be on guard when you pick up your pen...

Anything you write can subject you to a liable suit, so the first rule is simple - don't lie! You can never be held liable if your speaking the truth. As far as defamation of character is concerned, one not only has to prove that this has taken place, but that these words somehow damaged someone - physically, monetarily, emotionally - somehow it had to do harm. In conjunction with maintaining this journalistic integrity, document supporting evidence. People will take you more seriously if other authors support your assertions.

The next strategy fits right in with the first. If your commentary involves a certain institution, organization, or person, state your case without mentioning specific names. Generalize your subject matter to a more global issue, but still highlight your individual point of view. You could refer to this as "protective ambiguity." Begin a statement with the words, "over my twenty years of experience I discovered...," or I have worked at many institutions and have seen..." You can also use what authors term the "composite" story. Using this writing technique you combine elements of several similar incidents to portray the entire story. In this manner you protect everyone's right to confidentiality. While some may say this is a coward's way out, if you wish to present your case, you may have to resort to such tactics to avoid being sued. We do live in a litigious society.

Do not represent anyone other than yourself. Institutions can charge you are trying to use their good name to bolster your own credibility. They can twist this into conflict of interest, and state you were not authorized to represent the company. If your ideas don't reflect institutional interests management can then follow up with your termination - or possibly even file suit against you. Feel free to use all of your own credentials, i.e., R.N., B.S.N., M.S.N., CEN, CCRN, etc., just don't borrow anyone else's credentials - even accidentally!

Conduct your writing, or any other outside interest, as a separate business. Function in a true business capacity. Do not discuss your writings at your place of employment. Employers will be quick to jump on this one, and will accuse you of using company time to operate your own business - again a conflict of interest. If anyone asks to discuss your written works, simply state you'll be happy to do so off company time, and off company premises. If an administrator is ranting and raving at you for expressing your opinion in the local newspaper, instruct them you are not at liberty to discuss this totally independent business with them on company time. This is appropriate, and you can offer to arrange a meeting with your attorney if further clarification is required. The word "attorney" gets everyone's attention.

Finally, if you fear reprisal from your management through clandestine methods (usually their methods of choice) use a pseudonym when you write. My experience has taught me managers often employ subversive methods of retaliation in order to prevent being held liable for violating your rights. Editors are usually understanding if you tell them you wish to have your name withheld to protect you from this type of malicious persecution.

Keeping these strategies in mind, let's examine a few actual court cases...

In the case Rahn versus Drake Center (31 F. 3d 407 - Ohio 1994), Rosemary Rahn, a nurse at Daniel Drake Memorial Hospital, published a press release stating the patients at this facility were subjected to "reckless endangerment." Her charges of patient endangerment centered around new managerial policies which "have caused widespread discontent among their hospital staff which has created a high absenteeism, possibly developing a patient endangerment situation." This hospital did have major problems at the time and was trying to regain its accreditation and Medicare certification. Notice right off she mentioned a particular institution, by name, and made very specific charges against that institution - things which I have suggested to avoid. She was terminated swiftly.

Nurse Rahn brought suit against the institution for violating her right to free speech which was upheld by the U.S. District Court for the Southern District of Ohio. The hospital appealed, however, and the U.S. Court of Appeals, Sixth Circuit, held that the nurse's press release did not touch upon matters of "Public Concern" so she was not protected by the First Amendment. Here in lies the problem of publicly expressing your opinion about a specific institution or institutional problem. No matter how honest, or how valid, the issue, the law limits your protection from "wrongful termination" by requiring proof of public concern. Even in this case, there were dissenting justices which believed the matter in question was of public concern. Unfortunately for nurse Rahn, you must have a majority ruling. Had she not named the institution, and generalized the issue to one which could be affecting all health care institutions, she may have been able to state her case without fear of reprisal.

In the case of Willis Versus University Health Services, Inc. (993 F. 2d 837 - GA 1993), A nurse expressed her opinion regarding unnecessary C-sections, and traumatic births being performed by obstetricians for the sake of avoiding malpractice suits. In this case, the nurse generalized her remarks to "Obstetricians in Atlanta," however, once terminated and in court, the wrong defense was chosen. Her employers, after reading her article, terminated her for " loss of confidence due to poor judgment," and the nurse brought suit alleging violation of the Civil Rights Act, and violation of her First and Fourteenth Amendment Rights. While this seems appropriate, apparently she was unable to prove this was a "State Run" institution, even though it was contracted by the state to provide health care. It seems private corporations have more flexibility in firing their employees "at will" than state or federally operated institutions. Had the nurse argued the "Public Policy" exception to the employment at will doctrine, she might have fared better - hard to tell. Its easy to see that employers sure like to silence nurses from speaking out.

In another case, (Teeters versus Scott - 733 F. supp. 1279 - AR 1990), the nurse in question made an anonymous call to a patient's family to inform them of abusive practices in a psychiatric hospital. It seems after repeated attempts to work with management had failed, and an abusive behavior modification program was still being applied to the patient, the nurse took matters into her own hands. Once discovered, the nurse was suspended for ten days without pay, and placed on six months probation for her actions. In this case the U.S District Court for the Eastern District of Arkansas held the nurse's actions were constitutionally protected under the "public concern doctrine." You see, not all nurses lose in court.

Finally, I would like to present a case which occurred in my home state, Missouri. It seems in Missouri nurses have a bit more protection than nurses in some other states. In this state, the Nurse Practice Act specifically states the nurses have an obligation to faithfully serve the best interests of their patients. The nurses in my state are obligated to disagree with any practice which could place a patient at risk. We are required by law to question actions, such as an incorrect treatment ordered by a physician, which could be detrimental to a patient. Such was the case in Kirk Versus Mercy Hospital Tri-County (851 S.W. 2d 617 - MO 1993).

Pauline Kirk, RN, a charge nurse on the obstetrical floor, complained that a patient had been incorrectly diagnosed by the medical staff and was not receiving appropriate treatment for toxic shock syndrome. Being unable to elicit the proper treatment from the physicians, she complained to the hospital's Director of Nursing and was told to "stay out of it." Nurse Kirk then complained to the Chief of the Medical Staff who agreed with her and appropriate treatment was finally ordered - too late as the patient's untreated infection resulted in her death. Nurse Kirk was terminated for "on several occasions she made certain statements concerning the hospital, its staff... which were untrue and detrimental to the hospital... these statements exhibited a lack of support for the hospital and the medical staff." Nurse Kirk filed suit, and the Circuit Court ruled in favor of the hospital stating that no public policy exception to the employment-at-will statue had been violated.

The Missouri Court of Appeals, Southern District, Division Two reversed this decision, recognizing the State Practice Act required the nurse to object to such bad medical practice, and further noted the nurse could have faced disciplinary action by the State Board of Nursing if she had ignored the improper treatment by the physicians. If the nurse had remained silent she could have been viewed as being incompetent, or negligent. Let's here it for Missouri for this is a state where nurses are required to speak out - employers beware - harassment is not welcome in this state.

I believe nurses need to become more vocal if they are going to confront, and help solve, the problems facing health care today. Nurses need to protest poor working conditions, poor salaries, poor benefits, poor equipment, and dangerous staffing levels. Nurses need to speak up when malpractice and negligence occurs, and protect their patients from the dangers inherit in health care institutions. Nurses must add their voices to the political front to achieve safe, affordable health care for everyone in this nation. But nurses must also feel free to raise their voices without fear of employer retaliation.

As a final strategy for publishing health care concerns I offer the disclaimer. In fact I will illustrate the appropriate usage of this strategy...

The author wishes to express the strategies out-lined in this article are helpful for avoiding employer harassment. The author is by no means an attorney, and is not, for a moment, attempting to provide legal advice. The author further wishes to state that the incidents of employer harassment described in his article could have occurred at any time over his twenty plus year career. These events could have taken place at any of the five hospitals, two nursing homes, three blood banks, one laboratory, and two research facilities in which he has been employed. The events could be a composite of events which occurred at several of these various institutions.

The author is also willing to acknowledge he may have totally mistaken the efforts of such administrative practices, and, in fact, the managers involved may have viewed these situations as just attempting to be supportive of a wayward staff nurse. Ha, Ha, Ha... The point is, a disclaimer appropriately used can protect you from unwarranted repercussions.

10 Patients Profits & Power

** As you read some of the commentary ahead notice how the strategies I have described are employed. Nurses can take their message to the public, but they must exercise due care when doing so.

*****

Chapter 2

Healthcare Criminals
Published in the Columbia Missourian
November 13, 1995, page 4A.

In the time it takes you to finish reading this article approximately 2 million dollars will have been taken fraudulently from consumers by a new brand of criminal. White collar business managers and professional medical personnel pack their briefcases, or their black bags, with 11.5 million each hour from deliberate, coldly calculated, health care fraud. Our country spends $275 million each day for care which is unnecessary, inferior, never received, or for ghost patients which never existed. Total tab for fraud this year - $100 billion, or a full 10% of America's one trillion dollar health care bill. Over the past five years $418 billion, or four times the loss from the entire savings and loan crisis, was channeled into the pockets of these "healthcare criminals." We could have purchased medical services for all 40 million uninsured Americans. We could have avoided the entire debate on cutbacks in Medicare and Medicaid. But then again, mankind seems more crafty when it comes to stealing from each other than healing each other.

It used to be common to catch an occasional individual involved in healthcare fraud. A single physician or a dentist double billing Medicare - modestly exploiting the system. But when larger scams are perpetrated by institutions or conglomerates you're suddenly adding up millions and realizing this is a major criminal enterprise.

The reasons more criminals are entering the health care arena stem from lax oversight, dramatically increasing health care revenues, multiple hard to track billing systems, lack of coordinated information sharing between investigators, and an over-all poor system for reporting suspected fraud. Fighting fraud under these circumstances is about as easy as stopping the wind.

It is easy to hide your crime in a system of insurance based coverage. The average consumer pays only a portion of the bill directly, and understandably rationalizes how "at least I'm getting something for that premium payment." Consequently, consumers do not scrutinize their bills in the same manner as when they get their cars back from the shop. According to Michael Chertoff, U.S. Prosecuting Attorney, "Insured people don't have the incentive to find out if they've been over-billed and insurance companies can't audit every single bill." Under these circumstances, we become easy pickings for these illegal practices.

The FBI has 150 investigators who are currently processing some 866 cases of healthcare fraud. In addition to the FBI, the Health and Human Service's (HSS) Inspector General's office has its own investigative force attempting to process an additional 2500 cases of suspected fraudulent activities. With 1500 private insurers, and who knows just how many individual institutions and practitioners to monitor, it is clear these "health care detectives" are outnumbered, and once investigations are initiated it may take years before a case reaches a conclusion with a conviction, settlement, or dismissal.

In the most comprehensive "sting" to date the Department of Justice teamed up with HHS using a computer tracking system to identify some 4000 hospitals which falsely billed Medicare. Hospitals had billed for X-rays and lab tests on out-patients, and repeated the billing once they had admitted these same patients for additional treatments. The total cost to the American taxpayer - $100 million! If the hospitals in question refuse to pay back the money they will face fines of $5000 for each fraudulent bill under the Federal False Claims Act.

In my home state alone, 125 hospitals were included in the HHS crack down and they owe the government $655,000 from their false billing practices! They will not release the names of the hospitals, but just how many healthcare institutions do you think Missouri has - about 125?

This type of white-collar crime imposes tremendous costs on consumers who ultimately pay with increased insurance premiums, but these high dollar crimes still pale when compared to the ones which directly inflict injury on patients.

On August 25th of this year three former executives of C. R. Bard, Inc. were convicted for concealing information about faulty heart catheters. The company kept their cash registers ringing while ignoring health and safety laws and used patients as "human guinea pigs" to test their devices without FDA approval. The catheters frequently malfunctioned and broke during use injuring over 50 people and killing one Missouri resident. The company had paid $61 million dollars in fines, but finally, five years after the fact, John Cvinar, former president of Bard's catheter division, David Prigmore, former group executive, and Lee Leichter, former vice president of regulatory affairs were convicted of covering up their scam and could receive up to five years in prison and personal fines up to $250,000 each.

In another, almost unbelievable, case a pharmaceutical salesman was convicted of selling 6 million dollars worth of expired, mislabeled, unsterile, or previously used pacemakers over an eight year period. He was providing Hawaiian vacations and prostitutes as kickbacks to the cardiologists who agreed to implant the devices in unsuspecting patients. The Department of Health and Human Services even found a large number of bloody pacemakers in this gentleman's office raising suspicions he was re-selling devices surgically removed from patients or even from corpses!

There appears to be no limit to what these criminals will do to profit - even if it means injuring or killing patients! With additional confusion being produced by the growth of managed care initiatives and mega-mergers of health care companies, federal investigators expect the incidents of medical fraud and abuse to skyrocket. In recent testimony, Louis Freeh, the Director of the FBI, informed the Senate that even drug dealers are switching to health care fraud schemes as the potential to profit without getting caught is much better than from smuggling illegal drugs. He added, "Indeed, organized criminal enterprises have penetrated virtually every legitimate segment of the healthcare industry." Currently, very few perpetrators are caught so we can only imagine what other schemes are brewing. How will the ill and infirm be victimized next?

The best medical advice these days may very well be, "Stay well, and stay home."

Post-Script

While there is no question just how rapidly the health care delivery systems are changing we must ask if they are changing for the better. While the debate raged in Washington, business leaders seized their opportunity to restructure the system with only one thing in mind - profit. It was a perfect situation to exploit. Costs for care are growing ten times the rate of inflation and the consumer is demanding change. Managed care, under its various disguises, has effectively produced a massive shifting of dollars - away from institutions and professionals and directly into the pockets of administrators.

The next chapter provides some background - some creative ideas of how the industry could have evolved. It now stands in stark contrast with what has actually transpired...

*****

Chapter 3

Healthcare Reform:
A Revolutionary Nursing Perspective
*Published in **REVOLUTION** -The Journal of Nurse Empowerment*
Summer 1994, Volume 4, Number 2, Pages 40-44.

As we ushered in the new political climate of change with the Clinton Administration, we entered the decade of health care reform. We all know there is a crisis facing this nation in the way health care is delivered. We know 35 to 40 million Americans are without health insurance, and untold millions do not have access to basic medical treatment. We know national health costs are out of control - rising at an rate of 12 to 15 percent annually, and by the year 2000 will reach nearly 2.7 trillion dollars. We know the United States spent fourteen percent of its Gross National Product (GNP) on health care while no other nation in the industrialized world spent greater than ten percent. What we, the consumers of health care, don't know is how the "Managed Health Care Plan" which the Clintons have proposed is going to affect the profession of nursing - the core of patient care delivery in this country!

Physicians have always been the gate-keepers of medical access, and up to now hospital administrators have catered to their every whim in an attempt to maximize their revenue generating capacity. As the staff of Consumer Reports concluded, "the system is geared to providing the services that can earn physicians and hospitals the most money - not the ones that will do the public the most good," and physicians make virtually all the decisions that determine the cost of care, and the more doctors do the more they get paid." We can only hope that physicians are not truly stuck in adolescence, believing their "imaginary audience" is applauding their personal sacrifice to help the ill and infirm. The fact is, medicine with all of its rapidly growing technology, has become so complicated that physicians no longer know how to practice it in a compassionate and cost-effective manner.

Managed health care does little to nothing to correct this basic problem. It appears this type of health care system will create exactly what it preaches against - limited basic services, restriction of your choice of physicians to the managed care group in which you become enrolled, and a decrease in the quality of care as professional nurses, regarded as expenses, are replaced by technicians. In the article, "Healthcare Reform - How the System Works Against Nurses", Suzanne Gordon reports how "Managed Competition" has impacted the state of Massachusetts. This type of unbridled competition keeps hospitals bargaining to decrease expenses which unfortunately has become the definition of adequate nursing care. There also remains no incentive to curtail unnecessary procedures, tests, and surgery, but a strong incentive to cut the patient's length of stay in the hospital and the quality nursing care which they are entitled to receive. Competition, in this form, fosters volume versus need or quality. The net result of the Massachusetts plan has been to discharge patients too early without follow-up nursing care, and to eliminate hospital staff nurses at an alarming rate. Will this grow into a national trend?

These are but some of the many issues facing us all - not just the average consumer of health care, but also health care practitioners as they too will have to partake of the system created by these business mangers.

Nurses should become involved in lobbying efforts to ensure quality patient care is available to everyone. The following twelve points provide some revolutionary perspectives in how to attack our nations health care woes - expansion of nursing practice, appropriate restrictions on physician and hospital controlled practice, cost containment, and public disclosure of all available consumer information to allow the public to decide what services are appropriate for their care.

1. Treatment Algorithms: A multi-disciplinary team could put together standard treatment protocols for the majority of, if not all, medical diagnoses. We have used such protocols successfully for years in emergency nursing. Basic cardiac life support (BCLS), advanced cardiac life support (ACLS), pediatric advanced life support (PALS), and advanced trauma life support (ATLS) are all examples of this concept. Hospitals also have protocols for such diagnoses as spinal shock, drug overdose, alcohol detoxification, and emergency childbirth. All of these algorithms are tried and true methods of treatment which eliminate the physician practice of cover-your-ass (CYA) medicine. Standardization of treatment not only ensures that excesses will be limited, but appropriate treatment is rendered. These types of protocols can also be used as the basis for third-party reimbursement, as well as serve as the standard of care for practice. Any deviation from the protocol must be justified or absorbed by the institution.

Traditionally, physicians have argued their excesses in ordering treatments and tests are based upon their fears of malpractice litigation, however, the Department of Health and Human Services reveals this is a moot point in light of the fact the total cost of malpractice is less than 1% of total health care outlays. Furthermore, the Harvard University Study of New York Hospitals found only 3.7% of all patients experienced "adverse events" with 25% of these being related to negligence. Of the patients which suffered negligent care, only one eighth filed suit and only one sixteenth recovered monetary damages. The facts simply do not support the "technological imperative" of "if you have it you have to use it."

2. Regionalization of Health Care: Institutions performing a high volume of similar procedures with lower risk and less complications should be rewarded with more patients. It would be cheaper for national health insurance to absorb the cost of sending a patient to a facility where excellent care is provided as opposed to absorbing the massive costs associated with extended hospital stays caused by complications. This would stimulate competition for excellence versus maintaining the status quo.

There also needs to be some sensible limitations of services available, i.e. transplant centers. There is a major shortage of donor organs available for transplantation. The government, however, allows any institution meeting present regulations to go into the transplant business. Fledgling programs consume organs in riskier environments which would have otherwise gone to established practices demonstrating lower morbidity and mortality statistics.

Physicians and hospital administrators have made their positions clear - they have no intention of regulating themselves! In fact, the trend continues to be expansion and duplication of services through physician or business owned clinics, labs, and diagnostic services. These excess services are paid for by the consumer. When physicians are allowed to utilize self-referral for profit making, then laboratory work miraculously is doubled, and imaging exams such as CAT Scans and Magnetic Resonance Imaging are suddenly quadrupled.

Sadly, institutions are rapidly creating insurance plans to eliminate any scrutiny or limitations of these unnecessary practices. One hospital in my community just created its own managed competition plan which will force all of its employees to enroll for their services exclusively. To not sign on means you face a 50% increase in out-of-pocket expenses and a large premium increase. They also limit the services and frequency of those services provided - net result volume replaces quality. Increasing the volume of patients while at the same time cutting back the nursing staff (their expenses) will lead to disastrous consequences, but apparently patient care is a secondary issue when compared to the profits they will reap. It will be interesting to see how many of the staff physicians and hospital administrators sign on with the inferior plan they are creating. After all, they are the only ones making sufficient income to afford the more costly, but better, health care plans available in the region.

3. Independent Nurse Contracting: In the Winter '92 issue of Revolution: The Journal of Nurse Empowerment, Helen Borel's article, "Powerquake! The registered Nurse as Independent Contractor... The Mother of All Healthcare Revolutions" presents nursing with a sound alternative practiced by many other hospital departments. Our institutions contract out for blood banking, for specialty laboratory procedures, for laundry, for food services, and in times of staffing crises for agency nurses. Why not contract out for all of its nursing services? This would eliminate an entire hierar-

chy of parasitic managers which hospitals employ with the expressed purpose of exploiting staff nurses. We should be responsible for our own wages, our own benefits, our own continuing education, our own work hours, and basically take charge of our own profession. This would actually cut hospital costs while increasing our professional standing. Patients would, for the first time, receive an itemized bill which included a charge for professional nursing services. Patients would, for the first time, be able to place a dollar value on the professional nursing care they received, and be able to contrast that fee with other services they purchase. Patients would, for the first time, be able to see that nursing care is the best dollar buy you can get in health care today!

4. Cost containment for Physicians and Hospitals: There will have to be realistic limits placed on physicians and hospitals to prevent the wholesale gouging of health care consumers. There needs to be an acceptable standard mark-up at the retail level - say 300% as opposed to the present 2000% "if you can get it" attitude. Health care should not become another rich man's perk.

Why is there such a disparity in cost of care when comparing countries and institutions? Why does Magnetic Resonance Imagery (MRI) cost $1500 at a U.S. Corporate hospital, $1000 dollars at a U.S. University hospital, and only $177 dollars in a Japanese hospital? Why can a Canadian doctor perform a cholecystectomy for $350 when it costs an average of $2700 in the United States? Nations such as Canada, Western Europe, and Japan have adopted standardized pay schedules for their services through direct negotiation between physicians, hospitals, and government agencies. These countries have placed ceilings on expenditures to maintain fair prices for their consumers. Despite the negative publicity generated by special interest groups in this country, foreign health care programs are providing universal coverage which is fully accessible and comprehensive.

Again, managed competition may negotiate some price restructuring, but this will promote more unnecessary services as physicians attempt to increase the volume of their practice to compensate for any decrease in their fees.

5. Cost Containment for the Pharmaceutical and Medical Equipment Industry: It seems these big corporations are upset by any idea which could cut into their profit margins. If any form of cost control is proposed they threaten to restrict research and development (R&D) of new drugs and technology. Yet their own statistics show they only invest 12% of their financial resources into R&D while netting a 15% profit margin above the 25% return to their stock holders. These corporations are known to spend up to 25% of their revenue on marketing wining and dining physicians in an attempt to literally buy their prescriptive practices. Unfortunately, these tactics work as doctors commonly will order the most up-to-date and expensive products advertised when cheaper and effective alternatives are available. A classic example is Tissue Plasminogen Activator (TPA) used extensively for "clot-busting" in patients suffering myocardial infarctions (MI). This relatively new therapy is now used nine out of ten times in the treatment of MI, while streptokinase is just as effective, less likely to produce negative side effects, and only costs one tenth as much - $200 vs. $2000 dollars per dose. These companies need to focus on marketing what is best for the patient as opposed to what is best for their pocket books.

    6. Universal Coverage: There is no question that we must, as a nation, provide some form of healthcare coverage for all of our citizens. It is only prudent to limit costs in conjunction with this movement or else we will be creating a system which subsidizes wealthy physicians, hospitals, drug companies, and the makers of medical products.

    Whatever form universal coverage takes, it will have to be more efficient. According to the Health Care Financing Association, the present 1200 to 1500 private U.S. insurers are so overburdened with red tape that 14 cents of every premium dollar is spent on paper work. It is also estimated that hospitals spend as much as 25% of their budgets on billing administration so they can maximize their reimbursement from these insurers. A single-payer system, such as national health care insurance, would save 70 to 80 billion dollars in healthcare costs annually by streamlining the system of reimbursement.

    Presently the only federal regulation of private health care insurers is contained in the Employment Retirement Income Security Act (ERISA). Health care coverage was added to this 1974 piece of legislation as an after-thought, and instead of protecting the recipients of health care benefits it protects the employer's and insurance provider's rights to restrict, reduce, or completely eliminate coverage for anyone enrolled in their plans. This regulation does not require that employers offer health care coverage, instead it prohibits state laws from setting any minimum requirement for coverage. It also prohibits mandatory continuation of coverage if an employee becomes ill, and fosters discrimination against illness associated with race, sex, or lifestyle. Insurance companies faced with rising costs can raise premiums, raise deductibles and reduce benefits at will. Some insurance plans have simply dropped coverage for diseases such as heart disease, cancer, and HIV which can become costly to treat over time.

    The managed competition system practiced in Massachusetts appears to have magnified the choke-hold which insurance companies hold on reimbursement as they are virtually given total control to reject claims, deny coverage, limit referrals, and eliminate follow-up care in the home.

    Creating a national insurance program would not only ensure basic coverage for everyone, but it would allow portability and eliminate employee dependence on a particular employer. A single-payer national health care plan could easily be paid for by using the present system of employer contribution and employee payroll deduction. In fact, both parties would have to pay considerably less under this system to achieve the same level of coverage provided in existing insurance plans.

7. Increased Nursing Bedside Tests and Procedures: Nurses have always been the patient's advocate. Our efforts on the front lines controlling costs have been largely ignored purposely in order to propagate further patient exploitation. Nurses have performed bedside tests such as glucose monitoring for years - free of charge! Nurses have long used chemistry "dip-sticks" to test urine, tested for occult blood in patient's stool, and performed "spin-hematocrits" to determine if our patients were actively bleeding. Currently these tests have been striped away from our practices, and we have been told we are unqualified to perform these tests. Quality control has been used as an excuse to limit nursing practice in this area in order to increase patient charges. Fifty dollars per blood glucose, seventy-five per hematocrit, twenty-five per urinalysis, etc., etc., etc., all adds up to a considerable amount of money annually for the pathology department. Nurses can provide these services at a fraction of the cost while obtaining the results of these important tests in one sixth the time it takes for the laboratory to process the results. Hospitals have also refused to advance their technological capabilities in some areas as it would actually lower patient costs. A good example is a new device which would allow the bedside nurse to analyze a patient's arterial blood gases. A nurse could perform this test in two minutes at a cost of six dollars per test, but then again this would upset the respiratory therapy department which currently charges $100 for the same test and takes 30 minutes to perform.

Patients or profits? It's time for us to decide ... if we have the time! Managed competition has resulted in massive nursing layoffs already, so how long will it be before the remainder of us are asked to leave or face severe cuts in wages and benefits? There are 2.2 million nurses in this country who need to make their voices heard!

8. Empower Utilization Review: We have nurses and physicians walking around institutions documenting patient exploitation. These professionals call attending physicians and confront them directly with discrepancies such as leaving patients unnecessarily in intensive care units at a cost of $2000 per day - but nothing happens. Patients continue to receive treatment which is unnecessary. There is no accountability, and patients generally have no idea when they are being taken advantage of. Some process needs to be enacted to enforce utilization review.

The General Accounting Office (GAO) estimates a minimum of 10% of all health care dollars are taken from consumers fraudulently. Nation wide it was discovered that 53% of all inpatient days were not necessary, and 24% of all inpatients should not have been admitted in the first place! The 1990 annual survey performed by the Atlanta physician recruiting firm, Jackson and Coker, showed each doctor generated an average of $513,000 in inpatient revenues for the hospital where they practiced. It is easy to see why hospitals go to such lengths to recruit physicians by providing them top salaries, perks, and optimal working environments with the latest high-tech equipment, while nurses are regarded as expenditures which typically need to be cut at every available opportunity.

The Rand Corporation conducted its own study on unnecessary procedures and determined thirty-two percent of all carotid endarectomies were unnecessary. Fourteen percent of all heart by-pass surgeries - unnecessary. Twenty-seven percent of all hysterectomies, fourteen percent of all laminectomies, fifty percent of all cesarean sections, thirty percent of all upper gastro-intestinal exams, and sixty percent of all pre-operative lab work were totally unnecessary! All told, of the $817 billion spent on health care in 1992, $130 billion was paid for totally unnecessary procedures, tests and surgeries! In addition to all of this unnecessary medical intervention, hospitals, it seems, routinely over-charge patients by 5 to 7 percent on greater than two-thirds of their bills.

In contrast to all of this unnecessary expense, good nursing care prevents patient complications, reduces length of hospital stays, and saves money. So from an administrative point of view, it seems far better to keep nurses understaffed to impede the delivery of quality patient care. Expensive complications, after all, can be billed for. Nurses should be delegated to perform utilization review as nurses have no profit at stake to govern their decisions.

Managed competition promotes the exploitation of nurses for when cost containing measures are implemented under these programs highly paid executives protect their own positions and power by eliminating the front line care providers. It was reported on CNN that there are currently 1.5 administrators for each hospital inpatient bed - whether that bed is occupied or not! When have staff nurses ever enjoyed that type of staffing ratio to provide the care their patients require?

9. Published Price Lists: The most basic principles of a market economy are violated in the health care industry. Institutions and physicians should be required to list their prices so health care consumers can shop for their services. Competition in pricing is desperately needed in health care, and for those who might think such prices are relatively uniform, think again. In my community the private corporate hospital routinely charges double what the university hospital charges for the same care. Why should such variation be allowed to exist?

10. Published Patient Morbidity and Mortality Statistics: I can not think of anything more essential to judge your physician's skills than his or her actual record.

Health care practitioners have maintained a conspiracy of silence regarding this information. We are entitled to know if our physicians are truly healers! Granted, there are inherent limitations to some of these statistics considering the variations in record keeping and differences in patient populations, but consumers should not be treated as being ignorant and incapable of understanding such data. We should have a publicly available record of all doctor's practices for without public disclosure there is no motive, or pressure, to achieve excellence in the quality of care provided.

11. More Birthing Centers; Where else can nurses be better utilized to cut health care costs than in one of the most expensive areas of medicine today - child birth? Obstetricians charge some of the highest fees for services, perform the highest percentage of unnecessary procedures - C-sections, and all to earn an infant mortality rate of 21st among industrialized nations. Something is gravely wrong with this picture. Nurses have provided midwife services for centuries, and guess what is practiced in the countries with the lowest infant mortality? Certified nurse midwives safety manage normal pregnancies as well as, or better than, physicians, and their care reflects a lower incidence of low birth weight infants with shorter inpatient stays post-delivery.

12. Primary Care Nurse Practitioners: It is estimated only 30% of physicians enter family practice as compared to 50% just 30 years ago. The lure of big money in high tech institutions has removed doctors from the area of practice which can prevent the need for such high tech costly procedures. What better opportunity for nurses exists then to fill this gap in needed health care. One out of eight Americans has no access to a family doctor, and up to 33% of people residing in rural areas receive no primary preventative care. Nurse practitioners could easily fill this void at a lower cost, and save millions of health care dollars by preventing disease and costly complications.

It is unclear at this point just how managed care will affect nursing specialties such as midwifery, but strong lobbying efforts are in place by the American Medical Association to legislate strict physician supervision of all advanced practice nurses.

Simply eliminating the fraud, abuse, and waste in our present system would be a better start towards true health care reform as opposed to managed competition's efforts to limit services. These twelve ideas may help serve as points of discussion for formalizing a reform plan geared to providing quality patient care for all of our nation's citizens. We need to start somewhere! I believe it is time for nurses to represent patients in the political arena, the way we always have at the bedside, to be sure restructuring our health care delivery is true reform - not just a shuffling of health care dollars.

Post-Script

I mailed this manuscript to the White House in March 1993. I suggested choosing at least one bedside nurse to include in their discussion of health care reform. As expected, I received a "form" post card with stamped signature which essentially said nothing - not that I expected more, but it is clear those in power do not wish those on the front lines to have a meaningful say in what shape health care takes in the future. There is too much money and power involved to allow a common nurse, or any common citizen for that matter, to have a voice concerning such an important issue facing this country.

As we all know the Clinton Plan died in Congress in October of '94, but this didn't stop the corporate movement to take over the health care industry using managed health care as the blueprint for delivering services - or not delivering services. Now that the public is being given the opportunity to examine the fallout of such systems, perhaps it can renew the battle for quality care at a reasonable price. It will be a difficult fight against those with the power and money to buy legislative protection. And unfortunately, those in power are governed by the golden rule - the one which reads, "He who has the gold makes the rules".

*****

Chapter 4

Today's Shamans
Published in the St. Louis Post-Dispatch
January 5, 1995, page 7B.

Now that health care reform is temporarily dead in Washington, we have yet another chance to examine just how we want to shape this massive industrial complex. Just the mention of reform sends thousands of lobbyists, with millions of dollars, scrambling to buy off our legislators. Shouldn't this make us suspicious? If these special interests are willing to throw that kind of money away to maintain the status quo shouldn't we be asking why? Obviously, the people burning their money are trying to protect their future earnings from our illness and suffering. But just what has their system of profiteering off our diseases really done for us? How about a report card on how well our country is doing with the most advanced system of health care in the world?

David O. Weber, a health care journalist, has compiled a comprehensive list of health statistics in a recent article in Health Care Forum. After reading Mr. Weber's data, extracted from the Office of Disease Prevention and Health Promotion of the U.S. Department of Health and Human Services, one must ask if the doctors of today mimic their counterparts from the past - that is Shamans or Witch-doctors, rattling beads, blowing smoke, and taking credit when we miraculously get well. Here are some of the facts presented:

Babies born in 16 foreign countries have longer life expectancies than U.S. babies. The U.S. Ranks 23rd in infant mortality. American babies have the greatest chance of dying from an infectious disease or a parasite than all other developed countries. The rate of heart attacks, in the U.S. surpasses 11 European countries, Japan, and Canada. America is fifth in deaths per capita from lung cancer. The U.S. has the highest incidence of breast cancer in the world. One in 250 people in this country are infected with AIDS, giving the U.S. 40% of all of the AIDS cases in the world. The U.S. ranks fifth in deaths of pedestrians and motorists. Eleven other developed countries have lower death rates from cirrhosis and liver disease than we do. Suicide is the 8th leading cause of death in our country. Murder ranks as the tenth leading cause of death in this country with 2000 Americans being gunned down each month.

While these numbers are shocking even more shocking is that twice as many people die each month, as are gunned down, as a direct result of complications from medical procedures. That's 4000 people each month dying at the hands of physicians - not from their diseases! And every man, woman, and child paid out an average $4000 a piece for medical care in 1993 - who knows what that figure will be in 1994 and beyond? Is this what the American people have bought - snake oil, beads, and smoke?

Well not all of Mr. Weber's report card was bad. It seems that over the past decade we have added about 3.5 years to our life expectancy. However, clinical innovations have not accounted for any of this gain. We, as a society, have accomplished this increase in life on our own by eating better, exercising more, quitting smoking, reducing our alcohol intake, driving slower, wearing seat belts, protecting ourselves from sexually transmitted diseases, vaccinating our children, and dodging bullets in the streets. It sounds as though we need to add another element to our list of health promotion strategies, namely, more control over the procedures which health care professionals seek to inflict upon us.

We need to truly be receiving "informed consent", and obtaining second and third opinions. We need true competition in the medical industry - thus published price lists and morbidity and mortality statistics. We should be allowed to shop for the best doctor, and the best price, just like every other service sector in our society. Hospital administrators are now referring to patient care as being a product, and employees are part of the product line. If they intend to deliver health care to us in assembly line fashion then we should have some say as to what product we wish to receive - mainly safe, affordable, legitimate practice.

So while the lobbyists do the Shaman's dance in Washington, D. C. - selling their snake oil of "fee for service", shaking their beads of "don't interrupt our cash flow", and blowing their smoke of "regulation is hazardous to your health" - remember they are dancing on us. Four thousand of us pay the ultimate price each month related to bad practice. How many die because they don't receive any care? And how many of us will be bankrupt by the costs of one major illness? We had better make some decisions of our own before Congress resumes its next session.

Post-Script

Nurses decided to join the dance in Washington, and on March 31, 1995, 35,000 nurses demonstrated by walking in unison down Pennsylvania Avenue from the Capitol to the White House. Never before have nurses, from all different practice settings, and from all over the country, united in this fashion to carry the message of safe patient care to our legislators. Nurses are perhaps the only true patient advocates remaining as the only bottom line they have is compassion.

*****

Chapter 5

After The March
Published in the Summer issue of REVOLUTION -
The Journal of Nurse Empowerment,
Volume 5, Number 2, Pages 15-16.
Join the REVOLUTION! 1-800-331-6534.

What do you call 35,000 nurses marching down Pennsylvania Avenue in Washington, D.C.? Well, the overwhelming consensus seems to be "A Good Start!" And, a powerful start indeed for this most historic event. Laura Gasparis Vonfrolio, R.N., Ph.D., publisher of Revolution: The Journal of Nurse Empowerment, called for this demonstration, and all of her planning, organizing, promoting, and informing paid off in a big way for nurses all around the country.

Despite the lack of enthusiasm and support from many major nursing associations and publications, (the guilty know who they are) staff nurses representing every state in the nation showed up to meet with their representatives and demonstrate their resolve for safe patient care. The excitement and energy were palpable as nurses from every imaginable practice setting marched shoulder to shoulder from Capitol Hill to the White House!

These nurses took time out from their busy work schedules, their families, and their business obligations to send a message to the country that current management practices to reduce the number of registered, professional nurses in hospital settings poses a major threat to patient care and safety. Many nurses put their jobs on the line as hospital administrators sent out memos either denying time off to attend the march, or promising termination for those nurses who did demonstrate.

But, the demonstration didn't end in Washington. Many nurses, unable to attend, showed their support by holding local demonstrations, or by rallying with colleagues at airports as they departed for the march. In Chicago, for example, the Illinois Nurses Association sponsored a rally which drew 200 more nurses into the streets. Pamela Towne, a representative of INA stated, "we were really able to increase public awareness of these issues."

This type of self-sacrificing behavior is not new for nurses. Nurses put it on the line each day for their patients, fighting bureaucracy to ensure their patients' needs are met. As Joan Swirsky, M.S., R.N., Editor-in-Chief of Revolution, stated in her speech before the demonstration, "Nurses are the last patient advocates in America."

Critics charged that nurses are only worried about their jobs, but the message delivered to Washington was clear - nurses save lives! The latest wave of medical horror stories appearing in the media will only be the beginning if Corporate America has its way and cuts RNs out of the health care picture.

Simply put, the more registered nurses at the bedside, the less patient illness and death. Patricia A. Prescott, Ph.D, R.N., quoting over a dozen current research articles, documents a 6 to 10% decrease in morbidity and mortality if the R.N. to patient ratio is increased. Hospitals with higher numbers of R.N.s demonstrate higher patient compliance rates with treatments and medications, and a significant reduction of readmissions from complications.

In a study of patient outcomes, Roma L. Taunton, Ph.D., R.N. discovered hospital units with higher numbers of RNs demonstrated significant reductions (approximately 33%) of nosocomial urinary tract and blood borne infections when compared to units with less nurses. These infections cause 20,000 deaths annually, contribute to another 60,000 deaths, and run up costs of over 2 billion dollars a year. Who says RNs aren't needed at the bedside? Her study also documented decreased requests for pain medication, decreased patient length of stay, and consequently, decreased costs for those patients.

Nurses have demonstrated the importance of their clinical skills in study after study - the march in Washington demonstrated nurses' resolve to ensure their skills would be available for patients who need them. And just what do hospital administrations think they can save by eliminating RN positions? Money, of course. The consultants of Magellan Management Group in South Bend, Indiana polled 103 health care executives to see how cost-reduction initiatives, most of which involve the layoffs of registered nurses, were impacting hospitals. Most were able to reduce their costs by an average of 10%. The problem is, these administrators are pocketing these savings while sacrificing the quality of care you'll receive in the hospital. Have any of these so-called cost savings been passed on to the consumer? The answer is not only NO, but it appears hospitals, by their own records, never needed these savings (profits).

Hospital administrators are claiming they must cut back RNs as they're in financial crisis. Their own statistics don't support this position! Forbes magazine documented a 23% increase in hospital profits in 1991, an 18% increase in 1992, and a 19% increase in 1993. Fiscal 1994 is expected to be a banner year for hospital profits.

As more patients have been forced into managed health care plans by their employers, HMOs are having trouble managing the windfall. With membership up 11%, and earnings up 25%, the difficulty lies with managing their profits. Alan Bond, Director of Treasury Operations at Health Systems International, Inc. in Pueblo, Colorado summed up this problem in the Wall Street Journal with his statement, "Our problem is what to do with the money that comes in, not whether we have enough cash." His HMO's revenue is growing by $500,000 a day forcing Bond to "hunt for new ways to park the money in Treasury bills, certificates of deposit, and other short-term investments." So, when does the profiteering end? How many patients and professional careers must be sacrificed in the name of greed?

Nurses have been faced with a systematic dismantling of their profession. Not only are they being kicked out of hospitals, and having their technical roles assumed by unlicensed, untrained assistants, but it seems the legal system has abandoned staff nurses, leaving them victims of abusive management practices. The Supreme Court upheld a ruling last year classifying nurses as supervisors which essentially eliminates all protection nurses had under the Federal Labor Relations Act. The ruling of the court also emphasized that nurses must serve the interests of their employers and not the interests of their patients - a scary prospect indeed! While in Washington, nurses demanded legislation to restore their labor law protection.

THE DUST SETTLES

So with the march, press conferences, and legislative meetings behind us just who emerged as true nursing leaders, and who showed their true colors of opposition against staff nurses and their patients?

Let's start with the American Organization of Nurse Executives (AONE). Not only did their leaders denounce the demonstration as "unnecessarily scaring the public", but it was also rumored they placed a call to the White House to warn the President the staff nurses demonstrating were "violent", and posed a significant threat to Mr. Clinton's safety. What nonsense! Whether or not they actually placed this call is irrelevant, but someone must have made some threatening remark. The perceived threat was great enough to require the demonstration's organizers to be brought in for FBI background checks. Whomever perpetrated these tactics of harassment only further polarized the group's commitment to get their message to the public.

The American Hospital Association, and their affiliated state hospital associations, went on the offensive. Memos were circulated planning media coverage to discredit the demonstrators. Paid advertisements appeared in the press to highlight the role of technicians in hospitals, while minimizing the role of RNs. Nursing administrators were encouraged to select RNs, who could mimic administrative philosophy, to serve as media spokespersons, and thus discredit their own colleagues. Massive amounts of money are being spent to convince the American public that taking RNs away from patients will not jeopardize their care.

Where was the American Nurses Association? Well, the ANA did join the effort, but it appeared it only did so after realizing a major demonstration was coming to Washington and not participating would have been an embarrassment. The ANA provided some advertising, some bus transportation to the march, porta-potties, and cookies at the end of the march - if you went by ANA headquarters. Were they seriously involved or simply dragged into the debate? We may never know for sure.

The president of the ANA, Virginia Trotter Betts, addressed the crowd at the pre-march rally, but she appeared to have prepared a speech geared for the wrong audience. After mentioning the ANA's endorsement of the Clinton Health Plan, and her concerns for staff nurses, the crowd started chanting "prove it, prove it, prove it..." I found it hard to believe the distinguished president of our national organization would still be supporting a program which had died in Congress months before, and a program which supported managed health care - the driving force behind the massive layoffs of registered nurses. Appearing stunned at hearing the crowd jeering, Ms. Betts began to echo the sentiments of previous speakers such as Laura Gasparis Vonfrolio, who had called for national guidelines for nurse patient ratios, and for public disclosure of nursing skill mixes in hospitals. Ms. Betts received a better reception after dropping the Clinton rhetoric, but I didn't get the impression she was comfortable being among this group of staff nurses - perhaps she has been away from the bedside too long to know what issues need to be addressed? And, while it may have been intended to be a "nice gesture," it was not so comforting to know my membership dues were being spent on cookies instead of real representation.

The staff nurses were the real heroes at the demonstration, and the strongest feeling described in Washington on March 31, 1995 was that of hope. Many professional nurses, having grown despondent with the pressures they face daily, stated that for the first time in many years they were hopeful about the future. With such a large demonstration of solidarity and union, how could anyone present not feel re-energized!

Nurses were also enraged! Enraged to hear what their colleagues have been enduring, enraged to see how corporations are placing profit above patients, and enraged to see how traditional nursing associations and publications have backed away from the profession to avoid the risk of losing corporate advertising dollars!

WHERE DO WE GO FROM HERE?

Now that we are all home, and the stories of the march are beginning to fade, how can we continue the momentum? Donna Gentile O'Donnell, M.S.N., R.N., the Deputy Commissioner of Health For Policy and Planning in Philadelphia offered some sound suggestions. "Nurses must wage their battles State by State," she stressed. "Identify which positions in your political system impact health care policy, and target these areas for control." "Nurses must learn the political system and get active in it - learn how to organize, form a PAC, get involved in lobbying, and learn how to attract the media spotlight." Coming from a twelve year veteran of politics, these are sound suggestions indeed.

We cannot afford to let our moment in Washington fade. We must become involved! Write your legislators, take our message to the editorial pages of newspapers, and unite the public behind us. It's the consumers of health care who will ultimately demand the improvements required to ensure their safety, so nurses must assume the lead roles as consumer advocates and educators. Possibly the best thing nurses have going for them is public trust - the public believes nurses. We are credible! We have no profit motive to taint our true desire of caring for others. In the coming months we must not only exercise all of our skills to ensure positive outcomes for our patients, but to ensure our own professional survival.

The Media: An Integral Factor In American Politics

The Nurse's March in Washington, D.C. generated the most news coverage of any nursing event to date. Not only were the major television networks present, but thousands of newspapers, and radio broadcasts picked up the story. Yet some nurses returned to their homes to discover no articles in their major newspapers, or only short pieces provided by the Associated Press. Why have nurses not been more effective in capturing media attention?

Linda Everett of The Executive Intelligence Review in Washington, D. C. pointed out that with 97% of nurses being female, some view nursing issues as being feminist issues, and thus do not support those issues by default.

Edward Chen of the Los Angeles Times believes part of the problem was so many demonstrations occur in Washington that the nursing demonstration was relegated to being just one more.

Spencer Rich of The Washington Post added that many people perceived the march as coming from "a group of self-interested nurses only concerned about their jobs." He added, "there was no major social issue presented."

As we can see, nurses need to become more skilled, and articulate when it comes to presenting our issues. My own personal sense of why nurses attended was to be patient advocates - to call attention to the issue that patient care and safety are being jeopardized by current trends in health care which, in essence, are dismantling the nursing profession. More important than this message itself, however, was our ability to communicate it.

Apparently we, as nurses, need to try harder, and become more convincing to the media. We need to enlist the aid of those who can get our message out to the public. There is no force in this country which can generate the impact the media can, and we do have a major social issue to present - nurses save lives, and nurses are being eliminated from health care to maximize profits! If we employ the same commitment we show our patients to winning over the media, we will enlist a major ally in getting our message out to the public, and it is the public which can wield the key influence over health care administration.

Post-Script

So as you can see, nurses have started to join the battle to ensure quality care for all of their patients. This march was the beginning step, a step towards uniting the actual bedside providers of healthcare in this country. For too long others have dictated the role of these professionals. It is now time for the staff nurses of this country to take control of their profession - to take it out of the hands of those who only care about victimizing the ill and infirm for strictly monetary gain. Be watching for the next demonstration....

*****

Chapter 6

Therapeutic Misadventure
Published in the Columbia Missourian July 26, 1995, page 4A.
Reprinted in The Columbia Daily Tribune September 24, 1995, page 3D.

When the space shuttle Challenger exploded, NASA's Mission Control Center referred to it as being a "major malfunction." When civilians were killed during the bombing of Iraq, the military called them "collateral damages." When our fighter pilots accidentally shot down our own helicopters in the "no-fly zone" they had become victims of "friendly fire." The terminology various industries create to mask their disasters is fascinating. Referring to individuals as nameless groups who experience some "adverse event" relegates human life to the level of statistical analysis. Even Joseph Stalin, the communist leader who ordered "blood purges" of tens of thousands of people in Russia to consolidate his power, observed this when he stated, "A single death is a tragedy; a million deaths is a statistic."

Unfortunately, the medical industry, dedicated to the altruistic pursuit of healing, has become no exception to this ritual. An error in medicine which debilitates or kills is termed a "therapeutic misadventure." The man in Florida who had the wrong leg amputated, the Michigan woman who had the wrong breast removed, the Boston journalist killed by four times the correct dosage of chemotherapy, the patient who was disconnected from his ventilator by mistake and suffocated - all simply therapeutic misadventures.

In 1991, the Harvard Medical Practice Study determined that errors in treatment accounted for the deaths of an estimated 180,000 people each year! This is the equivalent of three jumbo jets crashing and burning every other day! All toll, 1.3 million Americans are injured annually by medical treatments -in Stalin's words "a statistic." The individual identities are lost, the pain and suffering hidden, the curtain is drawn, and the industry somehow remains untarnished - its all in how you word your disasters.

The July 5th, 1995 issue of the Journal of the American Medical Association (JAMA) reported that 19.4% of all medical injuries were caused by adverse drug events (ADEs). Errors in physician's ordering accounted for 39% of these ADEs, with an additional 12% associated with the way they transcribed the orders. Incidents associated with nurses administering medications accounted for 38% of the ADEs, and the remaining 11% of the errors occurred when pharmacists dispensed the medications. Not so surprisingly, the physician authors launched into a "systems analysis" of these errors and determined it was not any one individual or group of practitioners who were responsible, but rather the systems under which medical practitioners work which produce the errors.

Complex health care systems inherently impede the communication of vital patient and treatment information. Lack of knowledge regarding the medications was the most common proximal cause of errors producing 22% of the patient injuries, followed by lack of information about the patient's status or underlying conditions at 14%. The remaining errors were caused by violating prescribing rules on dosage and administration, by "memory lapses," or by inadequate monitoring. The errors specifically committed by the nursing staff were attributed to excessive workloads, and lack of experienced nurses.

This analysis takes on a whole new meaning in this age of changing medical systems. If medical systems are responsible for creating environments which generate life-threatening errors, then one must consider how the present health care reform movement will impact patient care and safety. Nationally, the proponents of managed health care are attempting to create "generic health care workers." These so-called multi-skilled workers are non-licensed, minimally trained employees who are performing any range of medical procedures ranging from nursing, respiratory therapy, x-ray imagining, EKGs, physical therapy, and of course, housekeeping. The same person emptying the trash one minute is providing your nursing care the next minute. The replacement of professional licensed staff with low-wage "assistive personnel" is presently accounting for massive layoffs in nursing and support staffs. Ironically, such systems bear the name Patient-Centered Care because they are supposed to decrease the present fragmentation of services provided in the hospital - remember, its all in how you name your disasters.

The JAMA study also revealed that it was the nurses who intercepted 86% of all medication errors and prevented their occurrence. The pharmacy staff intercepted an additional 12% of the errors so the massive number of drug related injuries were caused by the 2% of errors which slipped through the system. Imagine, if you will, how many more errors will go unchecked, and how many more patients will be injured as hospital CEOs attempt to maximize their profits by cutting professional staffs.

A study conducted by E.C. Murphy, Ltd., a national health care consulting firm, compared the staffing structures of 281 general acute care hospitals in the U.S. and determined that hospitals which reduce their staffs by 7.75% or greater were more than 400 times as likely to show increases in patient morbidity and mortality. Patricia Prescott, R.N., Ph.D., a nursing professor and researcher from the University of Maryland, documented specifically that higher R.N. to patient ratios decreases patient morbidity and mortality by as much as 5 to 10%. While the statistics support retaining more professionals, institutions employing various managed care strategies have targeted professional staff reductions ranging anywhere from 10 to 50%.

There seems to be no question that errors will occur in medical practice. If the physician researchers are correct in their assessments about health care delivery systems accounting for increases in the numbers of these adverse events, then we all, as consumers of health care, had better take note of how present and future systems are implemented. Managed health care has attempted to apply the same assembly-line techniques used in the production of wood pulp to the delivery of patient care. As the statistics of "therapeutic misadventure" rise under these new "drive through" medical plans, let's not forget these casualties have names, faces, and families. We might even know some of these statistics personally.

Post-Script

Medical error is a major issue of the times. With advances in interventional treatments the increase in physician induced injury was inevitable, and with current business initiatives to eliminate professional nurses you can expect the numbers to grow. There will no longer be a check and balance system between nurses and physicians.

Keep in mind managed healthcare is the driving force behind elimination of professional staff. In the next chapter single-payer health care is examined in the context of how it would impact healthcare in my state. This will perhaps serve to exemplify how it could be applied to the entire U.S. Benefits versus costs, however, is becoming less of an issue than just costs all by themselves. Let's hope this country adopts some system of health care geared to actually caring for people for it appears to me managed care does neither - manage or care.....

*****

Chapter 7

Missouri Health Care - Let the Citizens Decide

Published in the Columbia Missourian on June 9, 1995.
Reprinted in the Columbia Daily Tribune on June 18, 1995.

When Missourians voted for their state representatives and senators, we didn't intend to be excluded from the legislative agenda entirely. Sure we have a representative government, but major issues of importance to all of us should not be left to just that representative body alone. This is the reason Representative Mary Bland introduced House Bill (HB) 50 to the legislature. This bill was designed to give all Missourians a chance to vote on the shape of things to come in health care for our state. Sadly, the bill was defeated last month 102 to 57, but more sadly, most Missourians did not even know this issue was being voted upon.

What was HB 50? It was a bill calling for a public referendum on "Single-Payer Health Care". This is not to say our legislators would have voted on such a health care package, it would have simply allowed all of the citizens of our great state to decide an issue which impacts each and everyone of us.

Over 700,000 Missourians have no health insurance of any kind, and hundreds of thousands of us lack adequate coverage. In fact, with the present costs of health care today, the majority of us are one major illness away from bankruptcy. Yet, due to the high-dollar pressures of special interest lobby groups at our Capitol, we are being steered in the direction of managed health care.

Managed health care appears to manage profit shares over patient care. Dividends for stock holders take precedent over referrals to specialists. Administrative costs of HMOs are on average 31% as opposed to traditional hospital settings where only 25% is consumed managing the business of health services. Obviously, as administrative costs climb there is less to be spent on actual services to patients. Joseph A. Califano, Jr., the former Secretary of Health, Education and Welfare summed up this situation in the New York Times recently when he stated, "managed care has helped make America's system the world's most expensive to administer."

Examples where managed care has gone astray include Florida, where the state adopted the concept of Medicaid HMOs, and profiteering off the indigent population became the norm. Sixty-seven percent of Florida's Medicaid dollars were financing wages and perks of administrative staffs while patients with serious illness were denied or discouraged from using services. California shifted 80% of all state employees into managed care systems only to find their costs rise to 19% above the national average. It also seems physicians have been receiving big annual bonuses for the least number of patients seen. So much for the concept that HMOs were supposed to focus on preventative health care.

In keeping with the old adage that "one man's trash is another man's treasure," the HMOs have a different problem to deal with - too much money! Alan Bond, (I know I've quoted him before, but his remarks are wonderfully revealing) Director of Treasury Operations at Health Systems International, Inc. in Pueblo, Colorado summed up his company's problem in this manner, "our problem is what to do with the money that comes in, not whether we have enough cash." With HMO membership up 11%, and profits up 25%, his HMO's revenue is rising by $500,000 per day forcing Bond to "hunt for new ways to park the money in Treasury Bills, certificates of deposit, and other short-term investments." It would appear that if health care costs are reduced under these systems the savings are passed off to the corporations, not the consumers of health care.

Managed care rations medical services by limiting your choice of physicians, limiting the number of visits annually, and limiting specialty services. In addition, nothing is done to provide access for the uninsured. The current trends in managed health care also include the replacement of registered nurses with unskilled technicians, so once in the hospital you'll receive second rate care so CEOs can receive first rate profits. Do Missourians really want Corporate America managing their health care?

A single-payer health system takes the profit motive out of the administration of health care. Administrative costs are predicted to drop to 3 or 4% once the 1600 different insurance agencies are dropped from the billing process. (The General Accounting Office estimates administrative savings would total at least 70 billion dollars annually if our nation shifted to a single-payer system.) You can chose whoever you want to be your private practitioner, and this physician is reimbursed from a State Fund composed of employer and employee contributions - the same way insurance payments are deducted only cheaper. Everyone would have portable health care coverage not dependent upon individual employers. Businesses would benefit as their contribution to employee health plans would decrease from the present 14% to 12%, and small businesses would pay even less.

The 52,000 member physician's group, the American College of Surgeons, has endorsed the concept of a single payer health insurance program. David G. Murray, M.D., the chairman of the organization, testified before the House Education and

Labor Committee that this approach would be simpler administratively and preserve the patient's choice of physicians.

If this type of health care plan does not suit the people of Missouri, fine. Give us all of the facts and let us decide. Give us the opportunity to vote on the major issues concerning our society. One gets the feeling that after campaign contributions are made by the big insurance lobby, the pharmaceutical corporation lobby, and the American Hospital Association lobby (Hospital Administrators Incorporated) that the people's opinions no longer matter to our legislators.

Ask for a copy of the roll-call vote. See what your representative voted for - was it for your interests, or theirs. Ask for explanations of why they feel we citizens are incapable of deciding how we wished to be cared for. Almost everyone I talked to had no idea they were voting on this bill - WHY? Its time our representatives decide to represent us, on this, and any other issue of such magnitude.

Of course, when it comes to health care, our legislators don't have to worry - we, the tax payers, buy their coverage.

Post-Script

Of course, this situation is not limited to my home state of Missouri. We know there is approximately 40 million people in our country without health insurance, and there could be as many as 80 million who are underinsured. One catastrophic illness could wipe these individuals out financially - for a lifetime or beyond. One car accident, one heart attack, slipping on the payment and breaking a hip - one wrong step in your life and financially you will be owned by a health care provider.

Wouldn't it be in the best interest of all of us to choose a health care delivery system with a focus on patients as well as containing costs? Managed care is only going to provide inferior care while placing more dollars in the pockets of administrators. With the costs of care continuing to rise, our country will ultimately end up with a single-payer system or a system where only the rich and privileged few will be allowed access to services. I guess it depends on your individual philosophy as to which direction you would like to see this profession take. Currently, those in power are ensuring the corporate take over of medicine, and I personally do not cherish the idea of consulting MBAs regarding my treatment.

The next chapter examines how these business executives have crafted their strategy to eliminate licensed professionals from the practice of nursing. If you want to cut costs and increase profits then strip the duties of registered nurses which require licensure, employ a group of unskilled laborers to haphazardly provide care, and then put a shinny label on your system like "Patient-Focused Care."

*****

Chapter 8

Patient-Focused Care: The End To Hospital Nursing?

*Appearing in **REVOLUTION** -The Journal of Nurse Empowerment*
Summer Issue 1995, Volume 5, Number 2, Pages 40-43.
Join The REVOLUTION - 1-800-331-6534!

Imagine the "Generic Hospital Worker". An unlicensed, minimum-wage, technician who performs patient care, housekeeping, phlebotomy, EKGs, portable X-rays, respiratory treatments, and physical therapy. Find it difficult to imagine? Well, your managers have not only dreamed this cost saving idea up, but they are actively pursuing its creation - at your expense. "Patient- Focused Care", and its associated terminology, is the disguise for implementing a program which will eliminate hospital nursing as we know it - and will eliminate many hospital nurses along with it!

Imagine a hospital without staff nurses, and you can visualize Patient-Focused Care. A hospital where the only R.N.s will be called "Patient Care Coordinators", will serve administrative roles, and will govern the actions of all unlicensed technicians. One, or perhaps two, registered nurses per general unit. Any errors of commission, or omission, and guess who buys a new career - you do! Managers are carefully shielded behind their desks. Do I have your attention? Let's proceed with a long range analysis of this profit-driven system of health care delivery, and let's evaluate it now - while there are still hospital staff nurses left to examine its perils...

There is no question that we have waste in the current system of health care delivery. Consumer Reports extensively documented that 20% of all tests, procedures, and surgeries were completely unnecessary. In addition, 10% of all medical costs were directly attributed to pure fraud - scams from deceptive diagnoses, falsified insurance claims, and kickbacks from dubious referrals - all acts of commission from our esteemed physicians. If this is not enough waste, another 10% of all medical costs were incurred from totally unnecessary paperwork - no not the bedside paperwork nurses perform, however unnecessary some of that might be, but rather the paperwork involved in billing patients. In fact, 20% - 30% of the average hospital's entire budget is spent on the billing process to maximize third party reimbursement. If these statistics do nothing to your intestines just think, we currently have 1.5 to 2 hospital administrators for each inpatient bed in this country, and administrative costs have climbed 180% since 1968. Despite the incredible growth in administrative staff, and expense, managers are screaming that the price of labor is too high! In actuality, hospital labor costs have dropped by 11% over the past two decades. Hospital CEOs have painted a picture of economic hardship while their profits were up an average of 19% last year alone. With all of the statistics of medical fraud, waste, and abuse readily at our disposal, why haven't these areas been targeted for "redesign"? Instead of true reform, administration's answer to streamlining hospital expenses appears to be the elimination of as many highly trained, highly skilled, and highly licensed personnel as possible. Why? Because top notched staff require decent wages and benefits, and quality has never really been the issue in this industry - an industry expected to top 1 trillion dollars in gross receipts in 1994.

Enter the consulting firms...

Once health care reform became the topic of legislators, it opened the doors for hospitals to cut indiscriminately under the guise of reducing costs to the consumer. The timing was right to bring in business analysts - the same analysts which make assembly lines more productive were now fully welcomed into the unpredictable, no two patients (products) are the same, industry of health care. Booz-Allen and Hamilton, Incorporated pioneered the Patient-Focused Care (PFC) concept. Remember, this international management and technology consulting firm services large corporations and banks - a far cry from the delivery of compassionate humanistic services. Other corporations and consultants have jumped on the bandwagon, and restructuring is in full swing across the country and internationally. I will have to say that some of the analysis of these corporations is very accurate, however their prescribed treatment for our hospitals' ailments could prove to be more fatal than the disease.

The objective examination of our hospital structure is accurate. Our inter-hospital services are fragmented, and centralized away from the patients' rooms. Patients frequently are forced to make multiple trips throughout the hospital for specialty tests, procedures, and examinations. There are multiple specialties, with territorial boundaries, which dictate which professionals may perform each discrete task. In large hospitals, greater than 400 beds, there can be as many as 2-3000 employees under 320 different classifications - some of which only have one employee in an individual category. It is easy to see how this patch-work system can create inefficiency. In three days time a patient may be seen by as many as 55 different employees (one study claimed as high as 300 employees), be transported 15 times for procedures, and have multiple duplication in examinations and documentation. In terms of labor dollars, some studies show that less than 20% is spent on direct patient care, 14% on scheduling and coordinating activities, 19% waiting for something to happen (structural idle time), 30% on documentation, and the remaining 17% on other "bureaucratic functions". Agreeing that we have structural problems which increase inefficiency in providing patient care, we must now tackle the question of how to improve the delivery of that care? This is the point where nurses, the professionals who value human life, diverge from administrators, the professionals who value dollar bills. In the corporate mindset, labor is the largest cost, and consequently receives the largest impetus for consolidation or elimination. Our ever expanding management rarely recognizes itself as a part of labor cost, and while consuming the greatest share of employee dollars per person, it attempts to reconcile the budget "from the bottom up."

Are there areas of change which we can agree upon? No doubt about it! There is no question that a simple reorganization of departments within a hospital would help to decentralize services, eliminate unnecessary transports, and cut back on lost time waiting for services to be delivered. On unit physical therapy units, portable X-ray machines, EKG machines, satellite pharmacies, "patient servers" with supplies located in patient rooms, and the grouping of similar patients on each unit are all positive examples of how changing the physical design can impact patient care delivery. Where the major divergence in ideology occurs, however, is WHO is going to provide WHICH services.

Corporate ideology seems to be based on one concept, and one concept only - reduction of staff. The newest concept in staff reduction in a hospital environment is to employ "multi-skilling and cross-training". Actually what this amounts to is "de-skilling" or stripping away professional boundaries, and the only way this can be effectively, and completely, accomplished is through "de-licensing" our complex skills. Think about it. Administrators are moving fast. They are creating college programs with the end result being "a certified multi-skilled health care practitioner." If you think their efforts stop there, think again. Employer groups are lobbying legislatures for removal of licensure requirements. So after fighting for years to expand our roles as nurses, to achieve reasonable RN/patient ratios, and to provide "total patient care", we are now witnessing the dismantling of our profession, as well as the professions of all other licensed or certified therapists and technicians. Ironically, managers state that this will elevate our role, and eliminate the so-called unskilled tasks which we perform. Those in administrative circles don't seem to understand that we chose nursing to be at the bedside, to provide both skilled, and unskilled tasks, to make contact with all aspects of our patients - this contact is where true assessment, planning, intervention, and evaluation evolves. Yes, I tire of the definition of the nursing process too, but it is an intuitive part of us, the part that makes contact, and the part that heals. The few of us which remain, after the slash and burn of PFC, will be restricted to directing the actions of robotic technicians, and keeping the assembly line running.

Having examined the master plan for de-skilling, de-licensing, cutting vast numbers of nurses, respiratory therapists, physical therapists, radiology technicians, phlebotomists, lab technicians, housekeepers, etc.; we must now proceed with examining the issue of quality. With elimination of such numbers of front-line patient care providers, just what kind of quality of care will we be delivering?

The so-called "substance" behind the drive for PFC has been the concept of "Total Quality Management" (TQM), also referred to as "Continuous Quality Improvement" (CQI). The terminology implies an on-going process of evaluation and adaptation to insure the quality of services being provided. The TQM/CQI types of management were modeled after Japanese systems applied in industrial settings. Examples of the earliest of TQM/CQI programs in hospital settings included Guest Relations, Shared Governance, and Quality Care - described by one author as having the "shelf-life of cottage cheese." The latest in the chain of "answer to all problems management" has been PFC. It's obvious that problems would develop when trying to apply a system of management designed for the production of wood pulp to the humanistic service of patient care, but let's examine their measures of evaluation.

Claims to success for PFC are as varied as the institutions which employ it, but some common data has accumulated. Average length of hospital stay for patients has decreased anywhere from 0.5 to 4 days, depending on the institution and the unit in which the patient was receiving services. Patient satisfaction is reported to be improved based on surveys indicating that patients perceived the decrease in the numbers of care providers as equal to an increase in continuity of care. Patients were also satisfied with the decrease in transports for procedures and examinations. Clinical indicators, such as rates of infection, incidents, and medication errors have been reported to be lower - no objective figures cited. Physicians were satisfied that their patients were receiving as good, or better care on PFC units, and appreciated the relative proximity of services for patients, i.e. EKGs, x-rays, etc. RNs and technicians have been reported to have increased their satisfaction, as "jobs are more difficult, more challenging, and more satisfying". One institution reported a reduction in RN turnover from 33 to 19%, and another reported a "happier staff" as they saw a dramatic decrease in the use of sick time. Direct time spent performing patient care is reported to have increased, at one institution the increase was from 46% to 60%. By far the data which was most accurately calculated was the reduction in cost for the institution. Elimination of 10% to 20% of the workforce added up to an appreciable savings, and new supply patterns were calculated to save an additional 5-10%.

Part of the problem of evaluating PFC programs is that no two programs are implemented in the same way, but the biggest problems are discovered when one closely examines the data presented. Most authors offered general trends, and anecdotal reports - not hard data, and of the hard data presented just how accurate is it, and what variables were left out?

Length of patient stay is valued as a high quality indicator, but it becomes totally meaningless once you discover there is a corresponding increase in the amount of professional home health care required to complete the patient's adequate recovery. This data also totally ignored the advances in treatments and procedures, i.e. laproscopic gall-bladder removal, outpatient surgery, and community outreach services which lead to early discharge or kept the patient out of the hospital to begin with. PFC, in the studies presented, received all of the credit from extended outpatient services.

These same home health services greatly diminish the rates of readmissions for patient complications - complications which are incurred as a result of early discharge. I was only able to find one study presenting readmission rates, and this institution based all of its assumptions on reduced complications from one unit - the OB/GYN unit. One unit's figures hardly justifies a hospital wide program, and strikingly absent was a presentation of the actual numbers. It seems authors promoting PFC don't want us questioning the variables.

With regard to patient satisfaction, I discovered the biggest fallacy of all. According to Martin Strosberg, Ph.D. and Hans Lehr, MBA, writing in Quality Review Bulletin, the patient is left out of the process in determining what quality care is for them. According to these researchers, "Health care practitioners are used to making decisions they consider to be in the best interests of their patients, often without consulting them, they are also used to developing quality standards and clinical indicators without consulting patients." They further state that, "in industry, the consumer together with the manufacturer and/or service provider defines quality; in health care, the provider defines quality." And while I could quote their data forever, I'll stop with the final statement, "the direction of change must be driven by the needs and preferences of the customer, not the values of the provider." It seems in the complex world of health care delivery, patients are excluded from the process of determining what would be true quality for them. Rating quality based on the number of practitioners seen, on the quality of housekeeping services provided, on how fast a water pitcher is filled, or on the fact that you remained in one room during your hospital stay are not true indicators of the quality of the medical and nursing treatment which was received. Kicking patients out of the hospital faster is also no indicator of quality - especially when motivated by prospective payment systems. Managers know this all too well, and there still exists a real fear to teach patients what true quality care is, most probably because the number of malpractice suits would rise dramatically.

With regards to so-called improvements in clinical data, i.e. infection rates, errors, pt. falls, etc., I could find no collaborating evidence of such gains. In fact, at one institution in my community beginning to implement PFC, my nurse colleagues reported to me high employee dissatisfaction, and dramatically increased numbers of both patient complaints and incidents reports for errors - medication and otherwise. Patients, at this hospital, were asking, "Where is my Registered Nurse, I have not seen an R.N. since my admission." At this same institution, one manager's idea to reduce the time staff spent transporting patients was to have all ambulatory patients find their own way to other departments, such as radiology, for their exams. The net result was lost patients, bitterly upset by the apparent lack of concern for their safety.

As for the physicians rating patient care just as good or better in units practicing PFC, how would they know? Nurses know that physicians seldom read their notes. As long as bits of data, such as lab reports, EKGs, X-rays, etc. are spoon fed to them in a subservient manner they will always be content. For a physician to arbitrarily comment on the quality of nursing care is absurd. There is obviously a double standard here as nurses are never allowed to comment on medical practice - even if it kills a patient!

By the way, the institution reporting the "happier staff" based on reduced usage of sick time also had a policy in place whereby sick employees would not be replaced. This policy served as nothing less than a total coercion of staff nurses to come to work, sick or not, to prevent their peers from suffering yet more understaffing. To say that jobs are tougher, more of a challenge, and thus, somehow more satisfying is the biggest pile of garbage yet! Stressing staff, by preventing the delivery of adequate care, is not more rewarding! And the real reason nursing turnover is decreasing is because so many of us have been laid off that the remainder of us are clinging to our jobs for survival - no matter how poor our working conditions might be. Oh, how we can lie when it comes to the presentation of statistical data.

Lets back track a minute to the institutions employing PFC and examine the aftermath. In February 1992 the Healthcare Forum, a nationwide organization of hospital administrators, sponsored a conference - "Patient-Focused Healthcare Delivery: An Executive Conference on Strategic Operational Restructuring". This conference concentrated on the presentation of case studies of five hospitals which had implemented PFC on "Pilot Units." The Hospitals presenting were St. Vincent's Hospitals and Health Services from Indianapolis, IN.; New England Medical Center in Boston, MA.; Pacific Presbyterian Medical Center, San Francisco, CA.; Sentra Health System, Nolvolk, VA.; and Presbyterian Hospital of Dallas, Dallas, TX. All reported difficulties with implementing PFC. Ironically, all of the presenters indicated they believed that PFC was the only option to restructuring health care - despite their difficulties. One of the biggest problems cited was the high initial cost for the physical redesign of the experimental units. There is also a very high price tag demanded by the consultants directing the changes, but management felt these high costs were acceptable if the program would save money in the long term. Another major problem presented at this conference was the staff had difficulty "buying into it." No kidding! All administrators claimed that no one was laid off, employees merely had their job descriptions dramatically changed, or were relocated. Of course, there was some turn-over from attrition, and those staff members were never replaced. Nurses were particularly upset by the number of skills which they were expected to acquire, or direct, i.e. taking X-rays, and providing respiratory treatments, etc.; while at the same time experiencing a great reduction in their numbers. The remaining therapists and technicians found themselves as nothing more than "gofers." These highly trained, certified individuals were relegated to delivering supplies to the units where their jobs were being performed by nurses and aids. Obviously, staff morale, and job satisfaction diminished for all involved.

The question which arises here is whether or not this decline in morale and increase in attrition are just part of the plan of PFC. Attrition means "wearing down or weakening of resistance," and guess what, any employee who resists management's schemes is labeled "a force of resistance." Employees who resist are targeted for attrition, and the tools used to wear nurses down are referred to as "points of leverage." Our points of leverage include our salaries, benefits, vacation and sick leave, pensions, Holidays, and the biggest leverage point of all - STAFF MIX! Management manipulates your staffing mix, giving you less skilled personnel, and when you can not provide appropriate care, or even safe care, you burn out and move on. When nurses move on, due to attrition, they are not replaced, or are replaced with less skilled workers, which creates an even more stressful work environment leading to higher attrition rates. Using attrition as their most powerful tool, managers can easily change staffing for implementing PFC, and still claim that no one was laid off.

One of the biggest problems with PFC, which was not presented at the national healthcare forum in 1992, was the confusion and disruption caused by implementing this system. An example of such an experience occurred at Fairview Riverside Medical Centre in Minneapolis when American Practice Management, Inc. (APM) was employed to implement PFC there. Connie Curran, a former nurse and now head of APM, accepted a multi-million dollar contract to restructure their health care delivery to a PFC model. The changes proved to be so disruptive that another consulting firm had to be brought in to correct the situation. Maybe hospitals should cut costs by not hiring these types of consulting firms? Ms. Curran, of APM, was also contracted by several Canadian Hospitals, where she is affectionately referred to as the "bounty hunter." The nurses from the Manitoba Nurses' Union confirmed that with the introduction of PFC hospital costs were reduced — but at the expense of patient care, staff morale, and job security.

How did PFC receive such a positive spin in the first place? Reduction of cost was all that needed to be said to attract management, and with the providers dictating quality to their consumers they were sure to bias patient satisfaction in their favor. In his article "Well ?", David O. Weber, a healthcare journalist provides us with a little bit of reality shock. It seems that the U.S. Department of Health and Human Services, Mr. Weber's major source, cites the figure of 4000 people dying in this country every month as a direct result of complications from medical procedures. These people do not die from their primary diseases, but complications from their treatment. This is twice as many people as are gunned down in our violent streets each month.

There are over a dozen research studies demonstrating that nurses, at the bedside, reduce morbidity and mortality by 5 to 10%. The more nurses at the bedside, the less complications -it's that simple. Four thousand people die each month from complications despite all of the quality services which we have in place today. Imagine, if you will, what that number will be when management takes nurses away from the bedside. Imagine if you eliminate the highly trained, and highly skilled physical therapists, respiratory therapists, occupational therapists, X-ray technicians, laboratory technicians, pharmacists, etc., etc., etc.... along with those nurses. Health care has become specialized, and compartmentalized, because of its complexity. No one generic health care worker can possibly become an expert in providing all of these functions in any type of quality fashion. "You get what you pay for" say the makers of quality goods and services. If you somehow feel more satisfied to have one person take your X-ray, perform your EKG, deliver a respiratory medication, change your sterile dressing, mop your floor, and empty your trash, then go to a hospital practicing PFC. Imagine if you had generic physicians too - one which could by-pass your heart's clogged arteries, pin you broken bones, relieve that subdural hematoma, and master prescribing all of the 1 million plus different medications available to treat your condition - without any side effects or adverse reactions. Yeah right.

Prospective payment, or the reimbursement of medical expenses based on diagnosis related groups, has resulted in increasing patient acuity. Patients are not admitted unless severely ill, and hospitals earn more per patient if patients are serviced quickly. Ironically, at the time when hospital patients are more acutely ill than ever before, and are being discharged earlier than ever before, their care is going to be delegated to the least trained, least qualified, and least experienced breed of health care provider than ever before! Excuse my slang, but the concept of Patient-Focused Care is bogus. The problems are obvious. Patients are going to suffer, and many health care professionals are going to be sacrificed. What is PFC all about - its about profit.

Finale

A good example of how dollars interfere with the altruistic delivery of health care follows in the next chapter. Organ transplantation, perhaps seen as the most unselfish of all life-giving procedures, is subject to the same abuses as any other aspect in the healthcare field. In our country, if you have the money you can buy your position on the list of transplant recipients. Think not, well think again.....

*****

Chapter 9

Transplantation Can't Immortalize Heroes
Published in the Columbia Missourian on July 3, 1995.
Reprinted in the St. Louis Post-Dispatch on July 6, 1995.

Organ transplantation, normally considered a wonderful lifesaving measure, was suddenly thrown into the forefront of ethical controversy when Mickey Mantle received a new liver. Traditionally controversy has surrounded such procedures because of their high cost, their seemingly experimental nature, and their violation of various religious doctrines. However, the concern raised this time around was that of fairness.

The United Network for Organ Sharing (UNOS) was established in the U.S. to expedite the matching, procurement, and distribution of harvested organs. UNOS assigns a priority ranking based upon the patient's condition to ensure the equitable allocation of these scarce resources, but Mr. Mantle's liver isn't the first high profile case to start people wondering. A year ago the former Governor of Pennsylvania, Bob Casey, received a double organ transplant, a heart and a lung, after being on the UNOS list for only 24 hours. Mr. Mantle also waited only a day (average wait 3 to 6 months), but in addition some of his conditions, i.e. alcohol abuse, cancer, and hepatitis C, may have disqualified him as a suitable recipient at some transplant centers. Throw in a dose of wealth and fame, and that might lead some critics to call foul. Critics aside, the "Slugger's" real battles are just beginning.

Transplantation has never been the panacea which some believe it to be. The choice confronting the recipient of a heart, lung, or liver transplant may very well be a few more days versus the final exit - the only question is how long before the inevitable? End stage organ failure is an extremely devastating disease process whether self induced through alcohol abuse or caused by a mysterious virus or cancerous condition. While clinging to your own life you must await someone else's demise to get a second chance, and just how good are these second chances?

With a new heart you have about an 82% chance of surviving another year, a borrowed liver gives you a 77% chance, and a transplanted pancreas 44%. Kidneys and corneas survive that first year 90% of the time - the difference with these two tissues is the patient will not necessarily die once the new organ fails. In

Mickey's case, once his recycled liver dies, he dies, and the odds worsen after the first year.

Ok, a shot at another year is better than no shot at all, but once transplanted you must follow a strict and severe medical regimen. You must protect your new organ from your body's natural defense systems. Baylor University Medical Center has reported that our all-star Yankee is already experiencing a round of "light rejection". Cyclosporin, Imuran, Prednisone, Atgam, OKT3, Cytoxin, and ALS are some of the medications which Mr. Mantle may find himself taking to prevent or control rejection of his "gift of life." At an average expense of $30,000 plus annually you would think these high potency medications could work miracles, but brace yourself for the side effects. Not only are these medicines toxic to liver and kidney tissue, but they can cause high blood pressure, continuous headaches, continuous ringing in the ears, nausea, vomiting, and diarrhea. These drugs suppress the immune system to prevent rejection making even the most minor illness a life or death struggle. In fact, some recipients have died from the complications of transplantation quicker than had they not received their miracle transplant. Costs versus outcomes, risks versus benefits, is this whole process worth it?

The American Council on Transplantation reports the following organ procurement costs: kidneys $30-40,000; hearts -$80-140,000; combination heart-lung $130-200,000; livers -$135-338,000; pancreas - $30-40,000; cornea - $3,500 to $7,000; and bone marrow transplants can range $100-500,000. These costs typically include surgeon's fees, lab tests, transportation, and overhead. Not cheap procedures by any means, and one is left wondering why such huge institutional variances exist?

But back to Mr. Mantle and the issue of fairness. Considering the price ranges for organ procurement, scarcity of available organs, and Mr. Mantle's national prominence, one might imagine that profit or notoriety were motives in expediting his services. Surely we can trust the professional medical community on this one - even if 24 hours for a new liver is unfathomable. How would it be possible to be improperly listed in the UNOS system and receive preferential treatment? Personally, I'm glad Mr. Mantle received a new liver, and I hope he recovers quickly and as completely as is possible considering the limitations of such procedures.

Walter Williams, Ph.D., a professor of economics from George Mason University in Fairfax, Virginia suggests we could totally eliminate such controversy by opening a "free market" on organs. Somehow having organs available for the highest bidder, or if you're poor "mortgage your home," as Professor Williams suggests just doesn't fly well with me. One only has to look to India and Mexico to see the results of such systems of organ procurement.

In India, where everyone is allowed to sell their organs, the poor sell their organs to the rich, and this has spawned a thriving black market in human parts. Police in Bangalore recently uncovered a major network of "medical thieves" which were actually stealing organs from unsuspecting victims once anesthetized for other procedures. Lists of buyers in Turkey, Saudi Arabia, Malaysia, Singapore, and Europe indicated potential recipients had pre-paid for these organs!

At General Hospital in Durango, Mexico, officials are investigating how 61 healthy newborn infants mysteriously died. The bodies were returned to their parents with little explanation, and were found to have had their organs harvested. Perhaps organs and profits don't mix.

Our organ donation system may have its faults. It may even have hidden elements which influence the procurement process, but I seriously doubt we would wish to turn this portion of the medical industry over to the "changing winds of the free market."

Post-Script

Unfortunately for Mr. Mantle, he had one the most aggressive liver cancers known to physicians. Two weeks after the slugger's surgery the junior surgeon on his case admitted that his cancer was advanced, and they were unable to remove it all because it had wrapped completely around his pancreas. Mr. Mantle's prognosis was sealed before this operation took place. The senior surgeon dismissed the accounts of his underling by saying he had just not seen enough cancer to be drawing any conclusions. Another two weeks went by and low and behold the cancer had spread to his lungs and shortly thereafter he died.

Some say, bogus or not, Mickey Mantle's transplant drew public attention to the process of organ donation which may very well save some lives. A good spin, but as you can see by the physician's own data, transplantation is an iffy procedure at best. Throw in a little bit of corruption with how one acquires an organ and the public may just come to regard this whole process with a great deal of suspicion. And rightfully so.

Ever wonder why you don't hear more professionals speaking up about the immoral and unethical behavior which occurs in healthcare? (Ever hear this viewpoint on Mickey Mantle's transplant before?) Is it just the exception to the rule we hear about? Surely these medical horror stories are not commonplace? Well, I'm afraid our profession is full of such stories. They unfold before our eyes every single day. So why don't we see more about these topics - topics which should interest any consumer of health care?

52 Patients, Profits, & Power

Actually the public would hear more if nurses weren't bound and gagged. If we bring forth incriminating patient information we are charged with violating patient confidentiality and can be striped of our licenses. If we offer our opinions to the public we can be fired "at will" by employers. Nurses have been dis-empowered for decades by autocratic physicians and administrators, and any attempt at gaining some professional power has been met with fierce resistance.

In May of 1994 the powers-that-be got yet another chance to silence and exploit nurses. One ruling of the Supreme Court stripped away nurses' right to collectively bargain, and to advocate their patient's interests above their employer's interest. The next three chapters describe what happened and what nurses are doing to fight back.

*****

Chapter 10

The NLRB Versus Healthcare and Retirement Corporation
Is Anybody Out There?
*Published in REVOLUTION -The Journal of Nurse Empowerment
Volume 5, Number 1, Pages 48-49.
Join the REVOLUTION 1-800-331-6534!*

You don't recognize this title do you? Hello! This is most significant court case to impact the nursing profession in history, and where is everyone? Wake up! Perhaps you might recognize this if put in the context of the "Big Supreme Court Ruling". Now you got it, or do you? Lets start from the beginning....

When the National Labor Relations Act (NLRA) first passed, it allowed supervisory personnel to participate in collective bargaining and negotiate with their employers. Employers complained that not only did they have to deal with their regular employees, but there existed an unfair imbalance between labor and management by allowing supervisors to organize too. Well in 1947, after many lobbying efforts, management won, and the NLRA was amended to exclude supervisory personnel from the definition of being an employee (29 U.S.C., Section 152#). Congress defined supervisors as people representing the employer with regard to hiring, transferring, discharging, promoting, disciplining, directing, etc., etc... Congress gets long-winded. Back to the present....

At Heartland Nursing Home, in Urbana Ohio, four LPNs filed a complaint with the National Labor Relations Board (NLRB) regarding what they considered unfair discipline practices. The nurses had complained of deplorable working conditions, and were rewarded with termination - a familiar theme to some nurses. At any rate, the Board of Directors, of this corporation, contended that since the nurses participated in such activities as staffing, directing unlicensed assistive personnel, evaluations, and counseling that the LPNs were supervisors and not employees - thus not protected under the NLRA. The Administrative Law Judge reviewing the case stated that the nurses activities revolved around representing the interests of the patients, and not the interests of the employers, and ruled in favor of the LPNs. However, the

U. S. Court of Appeals, Sixth District, reversed the lower decision stating that the test for supervisor status was inconsistent with the statue. The Appellate Court then filed for a writ of certiorari (a review by the Supreme Court) which was granted. The Supreme Court stated that it was a false dichotomy to say that the nurses were serving the interests of the patients and not the corporation. Consequently, any nurse who uses independent judgment to direct the actions of any other employee (i.e. excuse me Mr. Janitor, but could you please empty the trash?) is a supervisor, and not eligible for protection under the NLRA.

Here we are, all dressed up and no place to go. Nurses no longer have any protection under any form of labor law or regulation. What about the ANA, and collective bargaining you ask? Well you can kiss the ANA good-by, because, as supervisors, we have no right to collectively bargain. Its not as though we will miss the ANA, however, for years their lame efforts have strengthened management and diluted the power of staff nurses - of course, that's just my opinion.

DePaul Hospital, in St. Louis, Missouri, is the next testing ground for this ruling. The staff nurses at DePaul just voted on unionizing, but management filed suit, claiming - you got it, nurses are supervisors not employees. The ballots have been impounded awaiting a decision.

So what now? Where do nurses go from here? Well there are two avenues I see for recourse. Active demonstration is a must. Not only do we need to fight for proper labor representation, but we need to be visible to the public. The public must be educated about what is happening in our profession. Patients must learn that the people on the front lines of their care are being abused! If we can get the consumers of health care behind us we will have more power for change - these are the people who pay the bills, and unfortunately money seems to be all that management understands.

The second approach which we can embark upon, is to try to de-supervise our positions. Yeah, that's the ticket. From now on lets not do management's work for them. Management can call housekeeping, can instruct our unit secretaries, can perform all of their own scheduling, and conduct all of the employee evaluations. Yes management can come to work and direct all of the unlicensed assistive personnel which they are using to replace staff nurses. Why should we participate in our own demise? If this is supervisory work, then let the supervisors do it. Or perhaps, we could continue to do the supervisory functions, but all of us would need to receive supervisory pay. Lets give all staff nurses a ten percent supervisory raise for performing all of those functions which makes us non-employees. What do you think?

Well I hope that you think something. Nursing is under siege! Our profession is crumbling before our eyes! We had better get motivated, and get tough with our response, because the alternative of allowing this continual abuse will not only be the demise of our profession - it will be the demise of our patients as well. Some day we will all be patients in the health care system which we are creating, if we don't choose the right path now it may be safer to stay home.

*****

Chapter 11

The Rise and Fall of the Nursing Union

Published in Revolution: The Journal of Nurse Empowerment
Summer Issue 1995, Volume 5, Number 2, p. 56-59.
Join the Revolution - 1-800-331-6534!!!

As restructuring of our health care system continues, nurses are being escorted out the door faster than ever. Layoffs for nurses are at an all time high. While managers speak the psycho-babble of their armchair vocations, replacement of professional staff with unlicensed personnel is escalating. Elimination of professional staff nurses will, according to management, translate into an opportunity for advancing our professional role as "patient care coordinators." What garbage, a "sanitation engineer" stills empties the trash. A "patient care coordinator" still follows the nursing process to intervene in all aspects of patient care - only now we will have more patients per nurse. We also know, if we direct all of the newly acquired unlicensed personnel, we will be held liable for their actions - or inactions. Our licenses are in increasing jeopardy, and simply because we are ruled by greedy administrators who value the all-mighty dollar more than compassionate, skilled nursing care. In light of these recent developments, nurses have turned to professional associations and labor unions for support only to find yet another rug pulled out from beneath their feet.

The Supreme Court ruling on May 23, 1994 effectively demolished the last staff nurse sanctuary which offered protection from abusive management practices. In the case National Labor Relations Board (NLRB) versus Health Care and Retirement Corporation (114 S. Ct. 1778 - OH 1994), the Supreme Court upheld a ruling by the Sixth Circuit Court of Appeals stating that the nurses fired from an Ohio Nursing Home were "supervisors" and were not entitled to protection under the National Labor Relations Act (NLRA). This ruling is far-reaching in its implications, for at a time when staff nurses are being forced to direct an ever increasing number of unlicensed assistive personnel (UAP), they have been classified as supervisors for this direction, and have lost all labor law protection because of their compulsory supervisory status. This leaves staff nurses at the mercy of "termination-happy" administrators during the most wide-spread cycle of hospital redesign facing this nation. Is it a coincidence that this major court ruling occurred just when hospitals were restructuring, and desired unlimited ability to indiscriminately put us in the unemployment lines? Who knows? One thing for sure, its time someone gave the ANA a "wake-up call" to let them know they no longer represent nurses. Perhaps they will be relieved, as they will no longer have to bear the criticism of not having represented us in a meaningful fashion.

At the exodus of this noble nursing institution, I think its appropriate to take a look back at nursing's labor movement. How did we arrive at today's impasse? Who have fought nurses during their battles for decent wages, staffing, and benefits? What glimpses of the future can we derive from administration's move to crush our representative bodies? Maybe we can gain some insight as to just how important it has been for nurses to unite with a common voice.

Many nurses traditionally opposed unionizing. It was looked upon as being "blue collar", or "non-professional." There was always the fear that striking, to obtain sane working conditions, would remove nurses from the bedside, thus not even allowing the provision of poor care. (There has never been a fear that management would voluntarily provide nurses with acceptable working conditions.) In addition, the employees of many state institutions and hospitals were forbidden by law to strike which undermined the power of unions to flex collective bargaining muscle. Labor laws, initially, were prohibitive and denied nurses the opportunity to form separate bargaining units. But nurses moved forward to consolidate their labor force, and gain additional leverage.

In 1974 the Taft-Hartley Act was amended by Congress allowing non-governmental, not-for-profit, hospital employees the right to unionize. The National Labor Relations Board (NLRB) had fought hard for these changes, and continued to fight for nurses to have the right to form their own separate bargaining units. Having an independent bargaining unit would allow nurses to concentrate on issues specific to the their own profession - as opposed to incorporating issues specific to other hospital departments such as clerical workers and housekeepers. As of 1991, the Supreme Court affirmed eight bargaining units per hospital allowing nurses to form separate units for collective action. Who do you suppose fought these changes which would favor nurses? You guessed it, the American Hospital Association (AHA), composed of administrators and physicians, have opposed any legal action which could possibly benefit nurses. This is why it took so many years, and court battles, for the NLRB to win us these rights. It's time for nurses to recognize just who their enemies are, and what they do to strip away their power. To understand the opposition all one has to ask is, why is the AHA so afraid of nurses organizing?

With health care costs continuing to go off the scale, and the public outcry for cost cutting, hospitals want to be able to freely cut nurses and nursing wages. Labor traditionally accounted for at least 60% of hospital costs, and nurses make up almost 50% of a hospital's labor force. A study of current statistics show that labor costs actually dropped from 67% of hospital expenditures in 1962 to 54% by 1992. In contrast hospital administrative costs have risen by 180%, and capital expenditures have risen by 36%. While RNs are being laid off, hospital profits are up almost 20% this year alone, and hospital executives have experienced an average 12% increase in compensation every year for the past ten years.

So while it seems that hospitals are making plenty of money, and hospital administration is making plenty of money, hospitals are lowering expenses by eliminating those of us who provide the direct care for patients. Eliminating expenses (nurses) has not translated into lower costs for consumers, but rather, higher profits for hospital administration at the sacrifice of quality care for patients. According to Webster's dictionary, a professional is someone who gets paid for their work, and while nurses do work in an altruistic occupation, and give of themselves in many ways, they deserve just compensation for their efforts. It would appear that hospital administrators have enormous resources from which to compensate nurses - if they were willing to do so. Losing the power of organized labor will make just compensation a very difficult issue to press.

After the 1991 ruling on separate bargaining units, and recognizing the growth in staff nurse resentment, management journals began advocating ideas to prevent nurses from organizing. Actually, most of the articles I read offered good suggestions. If you treated your employees with respect, open communication, retained your expert staff, provided nurses with the equipment and proper staffing ratios to care for their patients appropriately, and offered reasonable pay and benefits you would not have to worry about your nurses organizing and participating in collective bargaining. Not bad ideas, pay up now, or risk bargaining with a union later.

Despite these initial positive suggestions, nurses were becoming more interested in organizing than ever before. Why? While the journals were offering some positive strategies to eliminate the threat of unions, managers had been offering threats of their own. Management turned its back on the front line of our patient care delivery system. Instead of support, as the journals suggested, nurses continued to be told to do more with less, and put up or shut up. I wasn't shocked to read all of the suggestions to bust unions provided in administrative journals, but I was shocked to observe that managers were doing exactly the opposite of what was recommended to prevent staff from organizing. Perhaps they foresaw our unions' demise, because arrogance became the management style of choice. Apparently, administrators were not even concerned with the possibility that staff nurses could form a united front. They rarely, if ever, acknowledged that we could be strong enough to speak up for ourselves. Well, many nurses did mobilize to fight for better treatment, and for our patients' right to receive the care that only a nurse could provide.

So what did unionization produce for the nurses who successfully organized? Better salaries, wages, and benefits -approximately 6% better when compared to non-unionized nurses. Hospital administrators not only feared organized nursing for this reason, but apparently some "spillover" occurred. Once a hospital unionized, and the nurses received better compensation, the nurses at other area hospitals would receive better compensation due to the increased competition to attract skilled nurses. It appeared that administrators had good reason to fear us organizing as they actually had to treat us with a little bit of respect, and dignity. They even had to compensate us fairly for our services. Administrators are rejoicing the Supreme Court's ruling, and those gains in compensation, respect, and dignity have been shelved once again.

In all fairness we must examine the AHA's position on collective bargaining for nurses. After all, they contested that there were other reasons, other than maintaining the bottom line, for opposing unionization. The AHA points out that RNs with separate bargaining units tax the hospital system by demanding appropriate ratios between RNs, LPNs, assistive personnel, and patients. One argument put forward was that by allowing RNs to participate in such decisions they would be defining professional responsibilities for the various categories of health care providers. Nursing administrators have always wished to reserve the right to dictate our professional roles, and further argue if RNs determined their own roles it would create "competitive loyalties" between the other collective bargaining units when overlapping functions were divided. Time, and discussion to resolve matters of importance between professional groups, costs money which administration has been unwilling to spend.

The AHA was also concerned that simply negotiating with another independent union would be costly. They have deduced that contracting with all of the various hospital unions (8 bargaining units as supported by the 1991 Supreme Court decision) would result in the cost of approximately $360,000 for just one round of negotiations. Of more concern than this increased cost was the fear that RNs would demand some form of job security. This would eliminate management's ability to fire us at will, and it seems firing nurses is a convenience hospitals wish to protect - how else do you maintain an average 12% salary increase for administrators every year for the past ten years?

While the AHA has maintained their concerns did not center around cost, it appears that cost was their sole interest, and with the current legal ruling they can take comfort with not having to negotiate with us "bottom of the food chain" RNs.

Arguments concerning divisiveness among staff members never did hold up in light of actual events surrounding nursing strikes. In the Winter 1993 issue of Revolution, Dawn Chipman describes the nursing strike which occurred at St. Joseph's Medical Center in Joliet, Illinois. While there were many emotional issues involved, and their final contract may not have achieved all which the nurses desired, the nurses emerged with great feelings of camaraderie and empowerment. Other local unions offered to intervene on the nurses' behalf, and although the nurses did not approve of the other unions' methods, or accept the additional support, it disproves the AHA's argument of divisiveness between labor groups. Labor supported labor. It is more likely that the AHA was, and is, worried about dealing with a strong, united group of nurses who might actually demand what they deserve! The so-called high cost of negotiations was one reason unions worked - bargaining takes time and money, and with the dollar-clock running decisions favorable to nurses were forced.

If we want to be treated like professionals, have a voice in directing our practice, earn better wages, receive better benefits, and foster camaraderie and empowerment, I would have to conclude we need some form of organized representation. Yet we have now come full circle. Nurses fought the battles for over thirty years to gain separate bargaining units. Nurses resisted great forces of opposition to achieve job security, better staffing ratios, and better wages and benefits. Yet, in one swift ruling all of those hard earned benefits were lost. Hospital administrations have not stood by waiting for us to react, they immediately went on the offensive.

The nurses at DePaul Hospital in St. Louis finally attained a vote for a nurse's union in late 1994. Those ballots are now impounded awaiting a court decision on their right to unionize -brought about by their "supportive" administration. It seems the management at DePaul spared no cost in fighting the union. They were willing to spend over $200,000 to produce a movie, which they required all of their nurses to view, showing the AFL-CIO to be a corrupt union. They were willing to lose a multi-million dollar contract, providing health care to members of the AFL-CIO in St. Louis, just to prevent their nurses from organizing.

Providence Hospital, in Anchorage, Alaska, has waged war against their nurses for trying to unionize. At last check their ballots for a union remained impounded awaiting a decision from the NLRB. What ever the decision, you can be sure the administrators will pursue a conclusion in their favor.

Then we have Woodbury Nursing Home, in Nassau County, New York, where administrator Frederick White demanded his staff of twelve RNs quit their membership in the State Nursing Association or face dismissal. The nurses discontinued their membership in fear of losing their jobs.

At Michigan Capital Medical Center, in Lansing, Michigan, administrators simply canceled the election being held on forming a nurses union. It takes a great deal of effort to organize a ballot for union formation. A vote must be obtained requiring at least 30% of the representative group (thus the nurses) to agree upon having an union election. The NLRB then monitors the election. With hospitals preventing elections, or impounding ballots, nurses are not even being allowed the right to consider joining organized labor.

These are a but a few examples of administration's response to the Supreme Court's ruling. It has become clear what their motives are, and now, more than ever, nurses need to stop infighting and come together on the issues shaping their future practice conditions. Nurses need to become vocal! How else will our concerns be heard? We must lobby for an amendment of the language defining supervisors in the National Labor Relations Act so we can regain our labor representation.

It is our job to inform the public they may no longer be receiving the services which only a nurse can provide. Once the consumers of health care learn administrators are more interested in profit than in providing them with quality treatment, pressure can be brought to bear on hospitals to provide adequate RN staffing. After so many years of fighting to achieve decent working conditions, lets not lay down our arms and give up the battle.

*****

Chapter 12

Strike Back!
Published in REVOLUTION -The Journal of Nurse Empowerment
Fall 1995, Volume 5, Number 3, pages 56-60.

When the May 23, 1994 Supreme Court Ruling was handed down, classifying RNs as supervisors, nursing administrators believed their trouble with organized staff nurses was over. But as hospital administrators around the country try to play this "trump card," staff nurses are letting them know the fight is not over yet!

With the public appropriately demanding cost control in these times of skyrocketing health care expenses, hospitals are attempting to exploit nurses, yet again, to maximize their profit margins. The words consumer fraud come to mind as administrators apply the words "patient-focused care" to their schemes of laying off professional registered nurses and replacing them with untrained, non-skilled, unlicensed assistive personnel. And just who's costs are hospitals trying to contain? Employers are cutting their own costs in terms of both their own contributions to employee health care plans, and in terms of labor costs to deliver health care to the consumer. Hospitals, however, are not reducing costs which consumers pay for health care. Result: Consumers of health care pay more for less, and hospitals get richer - end of story.

Registered nurses are not sitting back passively while they, and their patients are being victimized. RNs, from Alaska to New York, are fighting back with the only weapon they have - unifying with each other. While hospitals are attempting to dismantle collective bargaining for nurses, RNs are digging in. Recent battles include...

The nurses of Providence Hospital, in Anchorage, Alaska, petitioned for collective bargaining, and the National Labor Relations Board (NLRB) ruled that almost all of the nurses, including charge nurses, were eligible for inclusion in such a bargaining unit. The hospital appealed in October, 1994, and a decision is forthcoming regarding excluding the RNs from collective bargaining based on the Supreme Court's ruling on supervisory status.

At the Greenlawn Facility of Michigan Affiliated Healthcare Systems, Inc., the argument put forth by administration was the same. The corporation tried to block an election for union establishment by claiming the RNs were supervisors, and therefore not entitled to protection under the National Labor Relations Act (NLRA). The hearing officer for the NLRB, however, disagreed stating, "the staff RN exercises authority which flows from superior expertise and knowledge rather than independent authority which flows from true management prerogatives." The NRLB ordered the representative election be held.

At Columbia Hospital for Women's Medical Center, Inc., in the District of Columbia, the Regional Director of the NRLB concluded the nurses did not meet the current definition of a supervisor, and their representative election proceeded on February 24th of this year.

While some nurses continue to fight just for the right to hold union elections, others, already united are taking their battles to the bargaining table, and if necessary to the streets!

The nurses at Sparrow Hospital, in Lansing, Michigan negotiated with administration to ensure nursing's input in staffing ratios to maintain quality patient care. The Michigan Nurses Association was able to secure a three year agreement creating a "Mutual Gains Committee," comprised of an equal number of union members and administrators, which will monitor, and approve, any restructuring plans the hospital may try to employ. They were also able to secure better shift differentials, raises in wages, and some protection in the event of layoffs.

In Florida, the nurses at Wuestoff Hospital took to the streets, using informational picketing, to keep the pressure on preventing massive pay cuts, and the elimination of educational differentials for advanced certification. They too emerged victorious!

The Illinois Nurse Association (INA) spent two years negotiating an unprecedented contract with the University of Illinois. With strong RN member support and an intensive grassroots campaign, the INA defeated what hospital officials had dared to call "Operations Improvement". Management's idea of improvement was the reduction of its RN staff from 88% of the skill mix to 65%. This reduction would have also reduced the RN's bargaining unit by a full 25%. While the University of Illinois was projecting a 6 million dollar savings with its plan, in reality their savings of 1.7 million were eaten up by having to employ agency nurses, at a cost of 2 million dollars, when patient care needs could not be met. The INA was able not only to reinstate the original number of RNs staffed, but added 80 RN positions to the University. The nurses obtained explicit language in their contract stating the RNs were not supervisors (avoiding the Supreme Court Ruling controversy), formed a Nurse Practice Care Committee to address issues regarding staffing, and attained a 3.5% raise in wages along with a 50 cent raise in charge nurse differentials. In addition, language was added to their contract restricting the delegation of nursing, and non-nursing, activities to the confines of the Illinois Nurse Practice Act, and only at the discretion of the RN as based upon her assessment. Finally, we get to the brave nurses in New York where two bargaining units let their administrators know, "they were mad as hell, and they weren't going to take it anymore"!

Mercy Nurses Keep The Faith!

The Nurses at Mercy Community Hospital, in Port Jervis, marched out on September 1, 1994 when the Board of Directors refused to ratify a union contract, and ultimately, to even acknowledge the union's existence.

In November of 1993 the nurses at Mercy held a representative election and voted in Local 1199 as their labor union. Contract talks began, but it soon became clear the administration at Mercy had no intention of seriously bargaining with their nurses. By August 19th, 1994 the union voted 3 to 1 to issue a 10 day strike notice. The purposes of such notification is so administrators will approach the bargaining table with serious intent to work out a contract, and also allow the hospital an appropriate amount of time to make arrangements for maintaining patient care should a walk-out occur. On September 1, 1994 one hundred and five unified nurses marched out into the streets to stand up for their rights to negotiate a fair labor contract.

Management had already made secret arrangements with U.S. Nursing Corporation, a company which specializes in turning nurses against each other, to provide replacement nurses for the strike. U.S. Nursing Corporation (USNC) makes immense profits from labor disputes providing travel, lodging, licensing fees, local transportation, expenses, and bonuses for nurses willing to cross the picket lines and dis-empower their own colleagues. While management was willing to pay the "big bucks" to their contracted strike breakers, they were unwilling to treat their own registered professional nurses with respect, and negotiate in good faith. By September 26th, 1199 filed a complaint with the NLRB alleging "surface bargaining," or no serious intent for management to settle the strike.

The administrator's strike breaking tactics really heated up as peaceful demonstrators were accused of "threatening and coercing" non-striking employees. One nurse on the picket lines was struck by a delivery truck, but not injured seriously. Was this an accident? Such non-sense was not going to dissuade the nurses of Mercy, some of which even joined a hunger strike.

Brenda Wolpert, an ICU nurse who participated in the nurses "Fast For Justice" for five weeks stated, "We will continue to seek justice and make sure the board of the hospital is held accountable for upholding the teachings of the Catholic Church (Catholic Doctrine supports organized labor), even if that means going all the way to the Vatican to see that justice is done."

Nurses also took their demonstration to the home of Thomas J. Moakler, Mercy's CEO, where they were met with a court injunction limiting their picketing to 2 hours per day, and 150 feet from his property line.

While the demonstrations continued, Mercy was watching the calendar, and when one year had passed without a union contract they circulated a petition to their temporary replacement workers asking for withdrawal of union recognition. This practice is illegal, and brought forth another NLRB complaint. Only permanent employees can sign such a petition.

Since the Sisters of Mercy in New York were contracted by Mercy Health Services in Detroit, Michigan, the union took its message to the workers in Michigan. When 1 million union workers threatened a boycott of Mercy Health Service's 15 hospitals, another injunction was obtained. This time a Michigan judge banned all TV and radio commercials supporting the union from airing in Michigan - so much for the First Amendment.

But Local 1199 pushed on relying in their faith in each other and in the Catholic Church. Catholic doctrine supports organized labor, and forbids permanent replacement of striking workers. The Sisters of Mercy heard the union's message, and the nurse's faith was affirmed when the Sisters appointed nine new members to the hospital's Board of Directors which then voted to support recognition of the union and proceed with contract negotiations. On March 2, 1995 a contract was signed granting the RNs a 4% increase in wages, no increase in their health insurance premiums for the duration of the contract, pension fund coverage, protection from layoffs for RNs with five years of service, and it provided a process to allow the nurses to have input into professional staff issues. Embittered members of the original Board of Directors are threatening a law suit. Terry Alaimo, Vice President of 1199 and chief contract negotiator, summed up these board member's continued resistance to settle the strike in her statement, "I never ceased to be amazed by the lengths some board members will go in order to avoid doing what is in the best interests of the hospital, the patients, and the nurses". As it turns out, several of Mercy's original members of the Board of Directors became so childish as to file a petition to remove the word "Community" from Mercy Community Hospital's name. After the Sisters of Mercy appointed new board members from outside the community of Port Jervis to settle the dispute, these physicians claimed the community's interests were no longer being served. It seems these physicians do not equate adequate nursing staff with the needs of their community?

Ironically, when researching the strike, Susan Bromley, spokesperson for Mercy, informed me the strike there was of little importance. Ms.Bromley added, "We are just a small community hospital being subjected to big labor tactics, if you want to follow a real nursing strike check on what is happening at Nyack Hospital, they had 450 nurses walk out." I can hardly conceive how a strike, the magnitude of Mercy's would not warrant coverage. A strike of six months duration, involving over 100 nurses, complete with hunger strikes, major labor representation in another state, and intervention based on Church Doctrine - not a story worth covering? Mercy's administrators obviously wished to steer me away from the embarrassing way they treated their nursing staff.

The nurses of Mercy are now back on duty serving their patients with the dedication of true professionals - professionals willing to fight for decent working conditions to ensure the highest quality of care delivery!

Nyack Nurses Unite!

Nyack Hospital, Rockland County, New York - nurses walked off the job this year with the major point of contention being the hospital's restructuring plan. Four hundred and fifty-one nurses strong, when these members of the New York Nurses Association learned their administrators were planning to eliminate their twelve hour shifts, and offer low raises, they demanded better! They began negotiations in January, but by the 29th of the month it was clear administration was not serious about bargaining with the nurses. In fact, the hospital had already blocked a union member from entering the building to speak with the staff, and had suspended two nurses for discussing the issues with doctors at the hospital. With the ten day strike notice given administrators contracted for 150 replacement nurses from U.S. Nursing Corporation, and began an advertising campaign claiming the elimination of twelve hour shifts would improve patient care.

With no common ground reached, the nurses hit the picket lines on February 7, 1995. Nancy Kriz, hospital spokesperson, tried to ease the concerns of the community stating the replacement nurses recruited from U.S. Nursing Corporation were all certified to work in New York. Kriz added, "It will be business as usual." Hospital Trustee, Paul Adler, disagreed stating, "I have never been in favor of bringing in replacement workers in any labor situation, I think it destabilizes the work force." Adler added, "The nurses (here) are probably the most valuable asset the hospital has."

Letters from patients poured into the local paper describing how they had preferred the twelve hour shifts, and felt continuity was better maintained with only two shift changes per day versus three which occur with eight hour shifts. Ironically, studies show an increase of errors occurring with changing shifts - more shift changes equals more nursing errors. Invalidating administrative claims further, the replacement nurses were hired to work the twelve hour shifts which managers were trying to eliminate to improve continuity! More frightening was the fact the replacement nurses would be working these long shifts six to seven days a week. With little rest, these nurses, unfamiliar to this institution and its patient population, would be expected to provide the same quality of care as maintained by Nyack's staff. It seems strike breaking takes precedence over patients, and its amazing just how much money these administrators are willing to throw at replacement workers while being totally unwilling to treat their own staff with any measure of worth.

Nyack hospital administrators are no strangers to controversy surrounding their restructuring efforts. The administration was recently forced to provide back pay and begin working on a severance package for the 60 LPNs it dumped in January 1994. The LPNs were replaced with nursing assistants to implement the concept of "patient-centered care." Now it was believed the managers, looking to replace RNs with unskilled aids, were trying to eliminate the attractive twelve hour shifts to drive RNs away from Nyack. This trend, to eliminate licensed nurses and replace them with unlicensed, untrained, non-skilled assistive personnel is growing in our country. Nurses have always "focused", or "centered", their care around their patients, and managers are using these terms deceptively to eliminate quality care provided by licensed nurses, and increase their profit margins by employing low paid assistive staff. By forcing unfavorable shifts upon nurses who had structured their family, educational, and occupational lives around maintaining these hours it was believed RNs would relocate to other facilities. This type of "planned attrition" would allow further reduction of professional staff, and replacement with lower paid unlicensed assistive personnel. Attrition has become the weapon of choice for administrators as highly skilled, and better paid, staff can be eliminated while avoiding the stigma of a layoff.

The nurses at Nyack proved their willingness to compromise, and an agreement was finally reached the first week of March. Lois Penn, the nurse's chief negotiator stated the, "Despite our continued concerns that the shift changes will compromise patient care, the union is yielding on this matter because we have become convinced the hospital administration is willing to destroy its nursing staff and the hospital itself to get its way." The union was able to limit the shift changes to 50% of the hospital's units, and appropriate time for transition will be provided as the hospital changes over these units to the eight hour shifts. Barry Waldman, a spokesperson for the New York State Nurses Association, expressed his hopes that "in the future perhaps the administration will consult with the professionals who actually provide the patient care before attempting to implement major changes which impact care delivery and safety."

Post-Script

The current "cut-throat" tactics being implemented by hospital administrators have resulted in a dramatic increase in the number of nursing strikes. The latest figures from the Federal Mediation and Conciliation Service indicate there were 27 nursing strikes in 1992 and 42 in 1993. If hospital cost-cutting strategies continue to focus on elimination of registered professional nurses, management had better prepare, for ultimately these profit-maximizing tactics will polarize staff nurses into a lean, mean, labor machine. Perhaps administrative greed will backfire and provide the driving force necessary to unify the 2.2 million nurses in this country - what a glorious thought!

Supreme Court Rules on Nursing's Supervisory Status

- Four LPNs working at Heartland Nursing Home in Urbana, Ohio complained to their management about deplorable working conditions in April of 1994.

- Management rewards the nurse's concerns with termination.

- The LPNs file an unfair labor practice complaint with the National Labor Relations Board, and an Administrative Law Judge (ALJ) rules in the nurse's favor.

- Health Care and Retirement Corporation, which owns Heartland, appealed to the U.S.Court of Appeals for the Sixth District which reversed the ALJ decision classifying the nurses as supervisors which excludes them from protection under the National Labor Relations Act (NLRA).

- The Supreme Court upholds the Appellate Court ruling on May 23, 1994.

- Legal definition of a supervisor: "Any individual having authority, in the interest of the employer, to hire, transfer, suspend, lay off, recall, promote, discharge, assign, reward,or discipline other employees, or responsibility to direct them, or to adjust their grievances, or effectively to recommend such action, if in connection with the foregoing the exercise of such authority is not of merely routine or clerical nature, but requires the use of independent judgment."

- The National Labor Relations Act (NLRA) of 1937 was amended in 1947 to exclude supervisors from NLRA protection when Congress gave into pressure from employers claiming an "imbalance of power existed between labor and management."

How To Become A Scab

U.S. Nursing Corporation (USNC) specializes in turning nursing colleagues against one another. In the Tuesday, March 7, 1995 issue of Newsday, Daniel Mordecai, the founder of this Denver-based travel nursing corporation stated, "We just do our business." "We don't get involved in the community."

Striking nurses at both Nyack and Mercy Hospitals strongly disagree. Vicki Soules, an RN striking at Port Jervis, summed it up in this fashion, "I don't believe you can call these people nurses when they're coming in here, taking our jobs and making so much more money for being a scab."

And money is at the heart of the matter. When you open the application form you receive from this agency its introductory flyer is printed on paper to look like money - specifically hundred, fifty, and twenty dollar bills. These companies must charge the hospitals they serve a hefty bill indeed as they offer the nurses employed $18 dollars an hour regular time, $27 dollars an hour overtime, paid travel to the city of the State Board of Nursing to obtain/renew your license, paid license fees, paid travel to the city of the labor dispute, paid lodging (at Nyack the scabs were lodged at the Hilton and given passes for free massages), transportation from the lodging site to the work site - if necessary, with special security personnel, on-site management assistance, weekly expense money (I received two different quotes - $235/wk and $435/wk), and completion bonuses of $2.00 an hour - usually an additional $1000. All told, the replacement nurse earns from $2000 to $3000 dollars a week, not counting the bonuses, and you know the agency charges more so they can earn a profit.

Why are managers so willing to pay this kind of money for replacement workers? It is obvious they're willing to go to great lengths to break the organization and will of staff nurses. Hospitals must be earning large profits indeed if they can afford to waste this type of money in attempts to exploit their workforce.

I strongly encourage nurses to stick together on labor issues, and boycott USNC and any other scab agency. Union nurses, on average, have 6% better wages and benefits than non-union nurses. Union contracts have forced non-union hospitals to raise their wages to compete. Management divides nurses by using manipulative tactics such as stating patients will suffer from union activities. These tactics only preserve hospital revenues, and dis-empower nurses.

Actually, it is a shame hospitals are unwilling to provide adequate numbers of professional registered nurses to care for patients, and that nurses must resort to collective bargaining to be treated fairly.

Steps To Collective Bargaining

- Nurses can identify an already existing labor group to affiliate with or create their own organization. Choosing a strong labor group, or one with large numbers of workers, is a valid strategy as larger organizations can wield more representative power.

- A representative vote must be taken of the group wishing to unionize. Thirty percent of the representative group (nurses) must sign cards expressing the desire for representation.

- The State Board of Mediation is notified, and the employer provides a list of employees for confirming the card signatures.

- The National Labor Relations Board monitors the union election which follows. Fifty percent plus one, of the representative group must vote in favor of the union.

- Once approved, negotiations may begin, but employers have no mandate to meet a time line for a completed contract and can drag the process out for ever.

- If no contract is ratified after one year, the employer can attempt to petition permanent employees to decertify the union. This requires the same 30% signature cards and another vote requiring a simple majority to decertify.

- It is a myth that unions can force their way into any organization.

Finale

While it's clear the labor force in the healthcare delivery structure has to fight for every inch of its influence just to take care of people under decent working conditions, those in power do little but bat an eyelash to generate a million in profit. As if this were not enough, corporations have resorted to illicit activities and just plain old-fashioned fraud to generate ten percent of healthcare costs. The following two chapters examine some of the devious way these companies pursue the all-mighty dollar.

*****

Chapter 13

Seeding, Misleading, Switching, and Stealing: The Vocabulary of Competition in Today's Pharmaceutical Industry

Published in the Columbia Missourian on July 12, 1995, page 4A.
Published in the Columbia Daily Tribune on July 18, 1995, page 7A.

Last month the Wall Street Journal reported that several pharmaceutical companies increased their donations to the GOP to influence legislation which ultimately saved them 1 billion dollars. It seems Abbott Laboratories, Bristol-Meyers Squibb, and American Home Products donated more "soft-money" to the Republicans this past year than the previous six years combined in an effort to eliminate rebates to the government from the sale of infant formula to the Women, Infants, and Children (WIC) program. Paying off legislators, however is just one method of dominating the pharmaceutical market, and these corporations go to great lengths to promote products which are much more lethal than infant formula.

Over $58 billion a year is reaped by U.S. pharmaceutical companies, but each individual company only commands a small share of this monetary battle field. Merck and Company, for example, controls the largest market share dominating only 6.2% of the industry. The fact that each drug manufacturer controls such a small portion of total pharmaceutical revenues fuels fierce competition to influence your physician to prescribe, or mis-prescribe, their medications. Dr. David Kessler, of the Center for Drug Evaluation and Research of the Food and Drug Administration (FDA) cites increasing evidence of illicit drug marketing practices which mislead or literally buy physicians' prescribing practices.

One such technique is called a "seeding trial." The company identifies physicians, not based on qualifications, but rather by their habits of prescribing competitors' products. These doctors are then enticed to prescribe a given medication by signing them on for a drug trial of no scientific value. Already FDA licensed, these drugs require no additional studies. The only criteria for participation is the physician's willingness to write prescriptions. Little to no data is collected, and no control groups are used to compare effects of the medications. The physician is paid a flat fee for each patient enrolled which usually varies from $85 to $500 dollars a head. Essentially, these false studies are designed to change a doctor's prescribing habits to a medication with no appreciable benefits for the patients involved. In a marketing memo intercepted by the FDA, one company highlighted the importance of one such trial in this manner, "if at least 20,000 of the 25,000 patients enrolled remain in the study, it could mean up to a $10,000,000 boost in sales."

This type of payment for questionable research has resulted in other problems. In his article, "Institutional Conflict of Interest," Ezekiel Emanuel, M.D., Ph.D. documented that institutions and physicians receiving royalties and payments associated with drug research were more likely to fail to provide informed consent; to ignore adverse reactions and complications endangering their subjects; and to introduce bias into the collection and interpretation of the data. Ultimately, we must ask if drug companies are eliciting false drug trials, and physicians are altering results based on payment for these studies, how can any patient trust s/he is being prescribed the correct product for his/her ailment?

If physicians can not be coerced into false studies to change their prescribing habits then drug companies simply misrepresent the benefits of their products. Unsubstantiated claims of superiority, minimizing or failing to mention risks and adverse reactions, or presenting pharmacokinetic distinctions with dubious relevance are all part of a well orchestrated false advertising campaign. A study conducted at the University of San Diego School of Medicine demonstrated that, at best, pharmaceutical representatives were only 89% accurate in their advertising statements. This 11% falsification of data could be all it takes for your physician to prescribe a lethal combination of medications.

If "seeding and misleading" can't get your physician into the manufacturer's camp then how about the "switch campaign?" Insurance companies encourage the use of cheaper generic drugs to hold down health care costs. To avoid this loss of revenue, however, pharmaceutical corporations offer direct payments to physicians to "switch" to another dosage form of the same product, or to another product in the same therapeutic class. No real benefit surfaces for the patient, but now there is no generic substitute for the switched classification and no loss of profits for the manufacturer.

If all of this doesn't make you reach for your antacid, then consider the newest trend in the pharmaceutical industry - stealing. Drug companies are trying to create alliances with insurers which will allow them to guide the patient's care, provide their medications, and bypass the physician altogether. A nurse would monitor the patient by phone while hospital and physician visits are discouraged. The drug company would provide only its products eliminating the physician's option to decide from a wide range of medications. I guess "stealing" prescriptive authority is certainly one

Seeding, Misleading, Switching, and Stealing:

way to eliminate the competition, but then again just who is practicing medicine here, and who's interest do you think these companies are representing?

In the November 15, 1994 issue of Hospital Practice, Dr. Robert Schrier documented a drug dosing crisis in America accounting for 60,000 to 140,000 unnecessary deaths each year. Adverse drug reactions resulted in 10.8% of all hospitalizations, 14% of all in-patient hospital days, and once hospitalized you have an additional 18 to 30% chance of experiencing an adverse drug event. Medications producing dizziness and sedation in the elderly population caused 32,000 hip fractures last year, and potentially life-threatening mixtures of medications were found in 88% of all elderly patients prescribed three or more medications. Prescription medications, taken the way they are ordered, account for more deaths each year than guns (35,000), than high-risk sexual behavior (30,000), or even motor vehicle accidents (25,000). In fact, each year prescription medications kill more people than the entire sixteen years of the Vietnam War where we lost 57,147 Americans! With these types of statistics, it is not very comforting to know that our drug manufacturers are illicitly influencing the way our doctors treat our aliments.

****

Chapter 14

Home Health and Medicare Another Fox in the Chicken Coop
Published in the Columbia Missourian on June 22, 1995

I was reading the June 5, 1995 issue of Modern Healthcare when I came across this advertisement: "As the Baby Boomers Get Older, The Profits Get Larger." The ad was placed by Staff Builders Home Health, and they boasted of thirty new franchises and doubling their revenues. Nice to know we "bommers", and for that matter all of us, are regarded as potential profits by these corporate health-care interests. I truly believe the words "health care" have been replaced by the words "profit shares" in this day and age, and it seems nothing is below these individuals when it comes to amassing wealth and power - especially when it comes to defrauding Medicare.

While Newt Gingrich and President Clinton were politely discussing how to control Medicare spending, many segments of the health care industry have their own plans in effect to "skim" Medicare dollars. One of life's little ironies I guess, but the same year we have the GOP demanding we cut Medicare and Medicare funds by $475 to $495 billion dollars over the next seven years we have the General Accounting Office (GAO) telling us that billions have been paid out to hospitals, physicians, laboratories, and home health companies related to nothing but pure fraud.

Medicare claims have jumped over 40% since 1989, and with so many providers billing the government tracking fraud has become difficult indeed. It seems this high volume of service can be easily exploited as illustrated by the "rolling labs" scheme where-by a single pathology lab obtains multiple provider numbers and then proceeds to bill multiple times for the same service pretending to be multiple labs. Some other examples of this massive rip-off include 2 billion in claims paid out which should have been paid by other providers, $170 million in over-billing by hospitals, and 5 million paid out to claims from companies not even enrolled for Medicare benefits. Double-billing is apparently a favorite scam, for if caught the perpetrators just claim it was a paperwork error and refund the money, if not caught the money becomes another payment on the boss's foreign luxury car.

Fraud runs deep in the medical industry, and the GAO and the Senate Special Committee of Aging estimate that out of our nation's total 1 trillion dollar 1994 health care tab a full 10%, or 100 billion dollars, were generated by illegal activities.

Over the past few years, one segment of the health care community has emerged from this cesspool of corruption to be in the forefront of defrauding the U.S. taxpayer - the home health industry. Medicare spending for home health increased from 5 billion dollars in 1992 to 13 billion in 1994 - a 160% increase! By the year 2000 home health is predicted to command 22 billion in Medicare expenditures alone. Medicare certified home health agencies have increased by 42% over the past four years, and this record growth tipped off the Feds that something might be amiss. Sure enough, investigators had no trouble uncovering illegal kickbacks, overcharging, ghost billing, double dipping, illegal referrals, unnecessary prescriptions, falsified patient care plans, money laundering, and racketeering!

There are currently eight major home health companies under indictment which collected revenues totaling $1.5 billion in 1994. With the government's estimate of 10% of those dollars being generated by fraud, $150 million dollars were taken illegally by these eight companies, $150 million which could have provided health care for people who needed it. Here are some examples of how these "caring" companies allegedly collected and spent our nation's health care dollars:

ABC Home Health Services, of Brunswick, Georgia, billed the American public for 800,000 in bogus claims including $5,133 to lease a car for the owner's son, $3,832 dollars for maid service for the owner's condominium, $2,831 for utilities for the condo, $3,263 in golf pro shop expenses, and $1,045 for country club fees.

Healthmaster, of Augusta, Georgia, laundered Medicare money through several dummy companies to the tune of 1.7 million. The company's top three executives now face a 133 count indictment.

Caremark International, of Northbrook, Illinois, was caught paying 1.1 million dollars in illegal kickbacks to Minneapolis physician David Brown. Other physicians affiliated with Caremark in Ohio and Michigan are now under investigation for the same "kickback for patient referral" scam. Caremark's defense is they didn't understand which business activities were legal and which were not.

St. John's Home Health Agency, of Miami Lakes, Florida logged five times the number of patient visits (1.1 million) in 1993 as any of its competitors of similar size. Once indicted for billing for nonexistent patients the company filed for bankruptcy.

U.S. Homecare, of Hartsdale, New York, appears to have forged nurses' signatures and other documents to create ghost patients. It just recently agreed to pay the federal government $650,000 to settle the allegations.

Beginning in October of this year the Health Care Financing Administration (HCFA) has proposed an increase of 20% in Medicare payments for capital expenditures, and a 1.5% increase for inpatient services. The Republican plan for fiscal '95 is to cut approximately $65 billion from Medicare which will undoubtedly reduce the number of persons eligible for coverage and the services provided. I might be totally off-base here, but doesn't it seem odd that more efforts are not being directed at controlling the waste and fraud in the system instead of debating how to direct and/or cut payments to legitimate recipients?

If the home health industry is any indicator of what is happening in other segments of health care in this country, our problem is not having enough resources to provide health care for everyone, but rather eliminating the fraud and abusive elements which waste those precious resources.

Post-Script

Caremark ended up paying out an unprecedented 161 million as a settlement for its crimes. The perpetrators walked as a result of legal council's ability to produce great confusion about what is legal or just simply unethical and immoral.

While these battles rage, nurses are being laid off in record numbers by administrators who chant they are too expensive to employ. Ripping off the ill an infirm through massive fraud doesn't compare to the fraud they are committing when they tell the public that professional nurses are no longer necessary to provide patients with quality care. Unnecessary and too expensive? Compared to what?

*****

Chapter 15

COMPARED TO WHAT?

Hospital administrators are putting forth the myth of registered nurses being too expensive to employ. Some even cast blame on RNs for increasing the already high cost of health care today - compared to what? Just as the grain in a box of cereal costs 5 cents when the box costs 25 cents (and you pay $3.50), nurses provide the true substance of patient care in hospitals for peanuts while managers rake in high profits to cast illusions of care and concern.

In an informal poll, and literature review, I collected prices of various medical professionals, treatments, tests, and supplies from around the country. Upon averaging these costs, and comparing, you will see nurses are the best dollar buy you can get in health care today!

The average RN's starting wage is $13.50 per hour. Twenty-four hours of highly skilled nursing care costs $324.00. The average annual RN salary is $28,800. What a buy when you compare it to...

- According to the AMA the average family practitioner earns $120,000.00 annually. Internists earn $130,000, cardiologists $250,000, cardiovascular surgeons $500,000, urologists $215,000, and radiologists $271,000. Some specialists earn as much as $2,000,000 per year! The average office visit of less than ten minutes of the doctor's time costs the consumer $45.00.

- The average hospital CEO in the midwest was earning $150,000.00 or $72.12 per hour. Managed care's highest paid executives throughout the U. S. averaged $500,000 in salary and $1,000,000 in bonuses. At $1.5 million total annual earnings these CEOs were pulling in $721.00 per hour. This still does not take into account various other benefits and perks.

- The average nursing administrator earns $70,000, or $33.65 per hour. Hospital administration has grown by 180% in the past twenty years, and manager's salaries are up 142%. Currently there are 2 administrators for each inpatient bed while floor nurses take care of 18 patients, and ICU nurses take care of 4 acutely ill patients. How many administrators do we really need versus the real people who provide your care at the bedside?

- A ride to the hospital in an ambulance costs $500.00. Helicopter services cost $1,000.00. It cost more to get to the hospital than it does for 24 hours of quality nursing care!

- The one second it takes to walk through the Emergency Room door costs $150.00 - the equivalent of half a day of nursing care.

- The average cost of lying in a hospital bed on a general medical/surgical floor is $700.00 per day. To lie in an ICU bed costs $1600.00 per day - this is just to occupy the space!

- The average cost of using the operating room suite is $1000.00 per hour. Your stay in the recovery room costs you $600.00 per hour or ten dollars for each minute.

- Being attached to a cardiac monitor for one day costs $250.00. It is the nurse who uses her expertise to interpret your heart's rhythm, and ensures you receive proper treatment from your physician. A pulse oximeter is charged at the rate of $150.00 per day, with the probe costing you $50.00. Again the monitor means nothing without the nurse to interpret it.

- If you end up on a ventilator during your hospital stay, add $900.00 per day for use of the machinery. That is three times as much as the nurse earns, and she performs much more than one simple function.

- Standard IV fluids cost an average of $50.00 per bag with three administered daily. IV medications can cost as much as $150.00 for one dose of an antibiotic (4 to 6 given daily), $250.00 a bag for TPN (3 required daily) to provide essential nutrients, $1000.00 for one bag of urokinase to dissolve a blood clot in one of your extremities (up to six bags required for 24 hours worth of treatment), and $2000.00 for a single dose of TPA to break a clot in your coronary artery! One dose of TPA costs as much as 6 days of skilled nursing care!

- Blood products such as one unit of packed red blood cells costs the hospital $350.00 for the processing fee - after mark up, it costs you $750.00. Specialty products such as fresh frozen plasma, platelets, and fibrinogen cost much more. Immune Globin, used for infections, costs $100.00 per gram, and daily treatment is 45 grams or $4500.00. Factor VIII, used by hemophiliacs costs 50 cents per unit, i.e. a treatment of 160,000 units = $80,000.00!

- Oral medications for a twenty-four hour period can cost from $150.00 to $300.00.

Compared To What?

- Laboratory tests can cost an average of $300.00 to $1000.00 per day, with simple blood sugar testing costing $50.00, and full chemistry panels costing $200.00. The same labs are commonly repeated several times a day.

- The average CAT Scan costs $1200.00, MRI is higher at $2000 to $6000 - add another $250.00 each for the radiologist's interpretation.

- A simple dressing change can cost $50.00, and a complex burn dressing may cost over $500.00 - these dressings are changed an average of four times daily.

While this study was conducted informally, and prices vary from institution to institution, you can conduct your own research. The next time you have to utilize a hospital's services, examine your bill closely. Scrutinize what it is you're paying for, and what in fact you receive. Ask what the hospital's ratio of registered nurses is to the number of patients each must care for. Ask if your hospital has been laying off registered nurses and replacing them with technicians. If it costs too much for your hospital to provide you with the care which only a registered nurse can provide ask, COMPARED TO WHAT?

Post-Script

While there is no question the direction corporate health care is leading us is towards an earlier mortality, some form of change in our present system is necessary. As the next chapter illustrates the status quo has produced a system of high cost experimentation. Unfortunately, turning health care delivery over to business executives will most probably result in even worse consequences.

The next three chapters examine some of the current systems in the industry which have, shall we say, "run amuck."

*****

Chapter 16

Has the Health Care Industry Crash Landed?
Published in Health Care: The Great American Hoax
March 1995

When a airplane crashes, and all passengers on board are killed, it's flashed across the country in a whirlwind of media coverage. What if three such jets crashed in the same day? And what if these type of accidents seemed to be happening with increasing frequency? We would shut down the airline industry until they met some type of acceptable standard for transporting people safely - right? Well in 1991, the Harvard Medical Practice Study determined that errors in medical practice accounted for the deaths of an estimated 180,000 people each year! This is the equivalent number of casualties from three jumbo-jets crashing and burning every other day!

The man in Florida who had the wrong leg amputated, the Michigan woman who had the wrong breast removed, the Boston journalist killed by four times the correct dosage of chemotherapy - this latest wave of medical horror stories has seemed to catch the public by surprise, while those of us working in health care can attest this is business as usual. As early as 1964, studies published in the Annals of Internal Medicine, by Dr. E. M. Schimmel, indicated that 20% of all patients admitted to university hospital settings suffered some form of medically inflicted injury. Of these injuries, 20% caused serious disability or death. By 1981, studies in The New England Journal of Medicine reported an increase to 36% of all inpatients suffering physician inflicted injury with 25% being serious or life-threatening. In 1989, a study presented at the 33rd meeting of the Human Factors Society by Dr. Gopher, in Denver, Colorado, showed that 1.7 medication errors occurred per patient, per day, in the medical intensive care unit. Twenty-nine percent of these errors had the potential for fatal consequences. Two years later in 1991, a study published by Dr. S. Bedell in the Journal of the American Medical Association revealed that sixty-four percent of all cardiac arrests in the hospital setting were not only totally preventable, but were caused by the inappropriate use of prescription medication. Moving on to 1994, Dr. Robert Schrier published an editorial in the November 15th issue of Hospital Practice entitled "The Drug Dosing Crisis". In his article it is revealed that 10.8% of all hospitalizations in this country are caused by complications produced by physicians mis-prescribing drugs - either the wrong medication, the wrong dosage, or in combination with incompatible drugs. Once admitted to the hospital you stand an 18 to 30% chance of experiencing an adverse drug event, and 14% of all inpatient days are generated by these drug complications. In all toll, 60,000 to 140,000 people die each year by following doctor's orders and taking their prescribed medications! The elderly are particularly at risk since 70% of physicians treating Medicare patients failed an examination on the proper way to prescribe medications to our older population. Complications, many life-threatening, occurred in 88% of elderly patients taking three, or more, prescription drugs. Prescription drugs also account for 32,000 hip fractures annually by making elderly patients dizzy or sedated!

What is going on? Why are we dying at the hands of those trained to heal us, and why are the numbers of us suffering the consequences of bad medical practice on the rise? With all of the gains in medical technology wouldn't you expect these types of medical casualties to be on the decline? Is this why the American Medical Association is campaigning for limitations on malpractice settlements?

Physicians are charged with the responsibility of diagnosing and treating our aliments yet autopsy studies show 35 to 40% of all patients are mis-diagnosed as to the cause of their deaths! A study conducted at Washington University School of Medicine in St. Louis, demonstrated that physicians could only predict prostrate cancer biopsy results with a 35% accuracy - a computer program predicted results with 87% accuracy. At Yale Medical School, a study of physician interpretation of mammograms revealed 20% missed diagnoses, 25% disagreement on treatment; and when examining the exact same cases 5 months later, 16% of the physicians disagreed with their own previous diagnosis and treatment.

Obviously, if a physician is unable to diagnose your symptoms and test results correctly, it is unlikely s/he will be able to prescribe the correct treatment or medication, and guess what, you become another statistic.

To be fair, some of these deaths are most probably the by-product of a combination of physician error, and the patient's pre-existing health problem, but the U.S. Department of Health and Human Services reports 48,000 deaths per year solely caused by complications of medical procedures! Whatever way you chose to look at it, people are dying at an alarming rate when they go to see their doctor. More people are dying in this country each year by following doctor's orders than are killed by violent crime (35,000 deaths), by high risk sexual behavior (30,000 deaths), or by motor vehicle accidents (25,000). In fact, more people are dying annually from medical treatment than all of these events put together plus all 57,147 deaths which occurred in the sixteen years of the Vietnam War! Isn't it ironic that with all of the accidental deaths which physicians cause, it is illegal for them to participate with assisted suicide.

If we need to ground our pilots of medical practice until their plane of medical diagnosis and treatment can fly, then by all means lets do so. After all, why should the transportation industry be held to a higher standard of care than our physicians? Perhaps now that we are gaining some insight into the health care system we can direct any reform movements to focus on improving the quality of practice instead of improving how physicians are going to be reimbursed for their services.

*****

Chapter 17

Physicians' Image Needs Healing
Published in The Columbia Missourian
August 31, 1995, page 4A.

In September of 1991 the Houston Chronicle began a series of expose' articles on its metropolitan for-profit psychiatric hospitals. The patient abuse reported was incredibly shocking and included "bounty payments" for patient referrals, insurance fraud, patient imprisonment, rape, and even one death. Two national chains and five individual hospitals were named with the Psychiatric Institutes of America (PIA) being the primary offender. One would suspect that after such negative media coverage the public would overwhelmingly reject these institutions, and any practitioners associated with them, when considering psychiatric treatment for themselves or a loved one. However, a study conducted by Betsy Gelb, Ph.D., Professor of Marketing at the University of Houston, demonstrated that public perceptions of these institutions were not significantly affected. It seems access to health care locally, just like our public utilities, is controlled by relatively few providers and healthcare plans so consumers seek treatment based on availability not quality. You take what you can get.

The headlines of 1995 have been riddled with similar medical horror stories. This plethora of reported patient mis-haps has shocked the general public and shattered our faith in an industry which we entrust with our lives. Human error, the inescapable equalizer, has produced medical mistakes ranging from missed diagnoses, to the wrong limbs amputated, to the administration of lethal doses of medication.

Perhaps the story gaining the greatest attention occurred when New York abortion doctor, David Benjamin, was convicted of second degree murder. It seems that after performing an abortion, and once complications developed, he simply walked out of his office operating room leaving his patient to bleed to death. He now faces sentencing of 35 years to life imprisonment for the death of 33 year old Guadalupe Negron. The prosecution aggressively pursued this case because it felt this physician was so "grossly negligent, and showed such depraved indifference to human life."

Dr. Benjamin's trial was totally unique, however, as doctors accused of malpractice usually only contend with a personal injury suit. Criminal charges are almost never filed, and actions against physicians' licenses are very uncommon. The American Medical Association (AMA) reports that 3 to 10% of our nation's physicians are either incompetent or impaired. Less than 1%, however, are disciplined annually. In 1994 for example 0.6% of U.S. doctors were disciplined, and a total of 1498 licenses were suspended or revoked. The reasons sited for these actions show it is rare for a physician to be disciplined for poor medical practice. Sexual misconduct accounted for the highest number of physician disciplinary actions, followed by substance abuse, insurance fraud, and prescribing medications to addicts in kickback schemes. The minuscule number of disciplinary actions for '94 did reflect a 12% increase in reprimands compared to the previous year, however, Gerald Bechamps, the President of the Federation of State Medical Boards, stated, "I don't think we're seeing an over-all increase in incompetent physicians, we're just doing a better job of finding those that are unfit to practice." Consumers of health care can only pray Mr. Bechamps is correct.

In the past it was easy for a physician to relocate his or her practice and leave behind records of negligence and malpractice. So in 1986 the National Practitioner Data Bank was established to track incompetent practitioners and help remove them from practice. This computer data bank holds information on any medical practitioner who is involved in malpractice litigation. Yet one of the AMA's stated legislative goals this year is to dissolve this tracking system, and block public disclosure of any information contained in these data banks. The AMA also lobbied hard to cap the amount of money which can be paid out punitively in malpractice suits. If all of their legislative activities succeed, the public will have to rely on physicians to police their own ranks.

So can we really trust our nation's practitioners? Well, in the July 1, 1995 issue of The Annals of Internal Medicine a study on the misrepresentation of academic accomplishments demonstrated that 30% of physician applicants falsified their credentials when applying for positions in the gastroenterology department at the University of Pittsburgh Medical Center. Dr. Harry Kimball of the American Board of Internal Medicine was quick to point out that while this individual study reported a very high rate of misconduct on the part of physicians in actuality only 7% of physicians nation-wide exaggerated their qualifications when seeking employment, and only 12% of doctors were deceptive in their Yellow Pages advertising. Seven, twelve, thirty percent? Should any such falsification of qualifications be tolerated? And, if physicians misrepresent their credentials to their colleagues and employers, what can their patients expect?

While consumers of health care usually accept whatever healthcare is available to them, the headlines of medical mis-haps are causing more and more questions to be asked. If the medical community is to regain our trust and faith in their ability to care for us then physicians need to heal their hemorrhaging professional image. Actions do speak louder than words, and presently it is the medical horror story which is commanding our attention.

*****

Chapter 18

Tobacco, Healthcare, and Politics
Published in The Columbia Daily Tribune, August 20, 1995, page 3D.
Published in The Columbia Missourian, September 8, 1995, page 4A.

America's traditional love affair with the cigarette appears to be officially dead, and two new criminal investigations being conducted by the Department of Justice have the tobacco industry running for cover. The legal posturing began when the FDA held Congressional hearings in April 1994 to consider classifying nicotine as a drug related to its potentially addictive properties. Charges of tobacco companies manipulating nicotine levels to ensure the addiction of smokers were steadfastly met with the industry's 30 year denial of there being any conclusive scientific link between nicotine, addiction, and lung cancer. The issue resurfaced this year when documents held by lawyers for Brown and Williamson Tobacco Corporation (B & W) were "stolen by a paralegal employee of the law firm", and reviewed by scientists from the University of California-San Francisco. A full thirty-two years ago, in 1963, an internal legal memorandum at B & W declared "We are, then, in the business of selling nicotine, an addictive drug effective in the release of stress mechanisms." In addition to confirming the addictiveness of nicotine, the 10,000 pages of laboratory data obtained showed that cigarette tar was definitely known to produce cancer in research animals.

Manipulation of nicotine levels and scientific data pales in comparison to other industry tactics to keep tobacco money flowing. Lobbying efforts have placed hundreds of thousands of dollars in "soft-money" contributions in the pockets of politicians - mostly Republican - to ensure a biased audience when it comes to regulatory changes. All toll Republican Party groups have received $4.7 million in contributions since 1991 compared to $1.4 million passed on to supportive Democrats. Need a plane to attend Newt Gingrich's fund raiser? Just ask U.S. Tobacco Company as 80 Republican House members did in June, and they will even kick in an additional $100,000 to dissuade current legislative efforts to ban sales of cigarettes to minors through tighter regulation. You also don't have to look far to find other prominent Republicans in the tobacco industry's pockets. Craig Fuller, Governor Pete Wilson's campaign chairman and top aid to former President George Bush, used to be senior vice president for corporate affairs with Philip Morris. M. B. Oglesby recently retired as senior vice president for governmental affairs for RJR Nabisco to join the ranks of Republican Party campaign strategists. Charles Black, republican campaign consultant, also represents Philip Morris along with former Republican Party Chairman, Rich Bond. Republican James Dyer, former Philip Morris lobbyist, is the current staff director for the House Appropriations Committee which one might imagine influences how much subsidy money flows into this industry of smoke filled death. With so much money, and influence, pouring into Washington one can only speculate what direction tobacco legislation will swing.

A recent survey conducted by the Robert Wood Johnson Foundation found that 79% of the public supported legislation to force tobacco companies to lower the nicotine content of cigarettes, and 74% favored banning vending machines to reduce minor's access to this known carcinogen. You might logically conclude the insurance industry would sign on with the public and support some form of regulatory effort. After all, 1000 people die in this country each day related to nicotine induced illness at an annual cost in the billions for healthcare expenses and lost productivity. Apparently moral logic and business don't mix, however, as it turns out the health insurance industry is one of the heaviest investors in the tobacco industry.

Prudential Insurance, the largest supplier of health insurance in this country, owns a large share in five of the six largest tobacco companies. Prudential's "piece of the rock" includes owning $100 million in stock of Philip Morris, $97 million in Loews (maker of Lorillard, Heritage, Kent, and Newport), over $36 million in American Brands (Lucky Strike, Carlton, and Benson & Hedges), $12 million in RJR Nabisco, and $44 thousand in the Brooke Group.

Prudential's investments aren't unique by any means considering Traveler's investment of $51 million in American Brands, and $37 million in RJR Nabisco. MetLife, not to be left out, owns $15 million in RJR stock. Cigna, another health care giant owns $57 million in Philip Morris and $18 million in American Brands. And, if ties between these industries aren't close enough consider the fact that William H. Donaldson sits on the Board of Directors for both Philip Morris and Aetna Insurance.

Conflict of interest? Apparently not. It seems this investment strategy is a win-win for these big corporations. Not only do insurance companies charge much higher premium rates for their smoking clientele, but investments in tobacco pay out sizable returns. These major players in the insurance industry have enjoyed windfall profits from the HMOs they own and tobacco, to them, is a very logical investment for this spare cash. Another portion of their profits are donated strategically to those same legislators taking money from the tobacco industry - an investment for future influence in how health care legislation will affect the sales of their favorite cash crop.

So why should we care if these companies profit massively from illness produced by tobacco? It would make sense for health care firms to have good health and preventative medicine as primary concerns for their investments. If executives simply pursue shareholder's interests to maximize their profits by selling us out, then one might also be concerned about other lobbying and investment efforts these companies are engaged in. Somehow using our premium dollars to finance lung cancer and shifty politicians doesn't sit well with me.

It is estimated that 1000 children are actively recruited to nicotine addiction daily by strategic advertising placed near candy counters, schools, and other shopping areas which children and teens frequent. Not much better than street pushers, the tobacco industry and its major investors have targeted our children for a future agonizing death so they may reap tremendous profit margins in the present. In keeping with the ironies of American business and law, wholesale death with powerfully addictive carcinogens is, of course, completely legal for adults, and when it comes to our children these money-hungry companies simply turn their heads the other way.

Post-Script

The old expression "Knowledge is Power" is definitely true. As the last three chapters have shown, a simple examination of our industry can be very revealing. So why the silence? Well, as I mentioned earlier, those in control of health care employ various strategies to keep us in our places. There will always be those who wish to silence us, and those who wish not to hear....

The next chapter is a lesson in malpractice. Not that any malpractice occurred, but the legal system didn't miss a beat when it came to profiting off of a patient's demise. And, where did the institution log in on this one? The hospital buried the story to avoid the publicity, and hung the financial burden, not to mention the stigma of professional incompetence, squarely on the shoulders of the defendants. Of course, settling out of court is not an admission of guilt - so they say....

*****

Chapter 19

Defensive Nursing
Published in REVOLUTION - The Journal of Nurse Empowerment
Fall 1994, Volume 4, Number 3, p. 43-45.

Four inches of fresh snow could not keep me away from my "appointment" at the legal building, but I found the reception inside to be far colder than this latest winter storm. I was there to give a deposition regarding a patient on my surgical unit. This particular patient had developed a mucous plug in his tracheostomy tube causing a respiratory arrest. Unfortunately for him, we only resuscitated his body leaving him with only brain stem function and in a persistent vegetative state. Unfortunately for me, I was the nurse in charge that night. No, I was not providing direct care for this patient, but yes, somehow I was responsible. Now I was about to learn just how nasty these matters can become, and just who would support me in this time of crisis.

I quickly learned what everyone was interested in - and it wasn't the truth of what had happened! The hospital attorney counseled me at length about what I could say and what I was supposed to forget - his interest being to minimize any impact on the hospital. "What ever you do don't implicate anyone else", and "just forget that the physicians were slow to respond to the code and acted improperly once they did arrive." "You can always say that you don't have any recollection of those events."

I was given some depositions to study, and told the hospital attorney would be right there beside me to protect my rights...

"D" day came, and the hospital's attorney was right there as promised. He watched the other side's attorney tear me to shreds without uttering a single word. After this grueling three hours has passed, he shook my hand and told me I had done all right and not to worry about it. I now understand what the other side was interested in too - they simply wanted to maximize their client's settlement. They were not interested in the truth either.

A couple of months had passed when I received copies of the depositions from the plaintiff's expert witnesses. (One of these experts, a doctor, went so far as to say that I, being an experienced charge nurse, should have taken control of the situation and instructed the physicians in what to do.) I was told to examine these depositions for any weakness in their arguments. This was an easy task. I prepared a twenty page report, citing twenty-five different references, which refuted every single charge brought forth by the prosecution. The hospital attorney did not even say thank you, and I learned later he had simply thrown it in the trash. No one was, at any time, interested in taking this case to court to bring out the facts. This was a well rehearsed legal dance about how much money would be paid to whom and by whom.

I had already informed my malpractice insurance company of what was happening, and they too assigned an attorney to keep watch over the hospital's attorney. I forwarded them a copy of my arguments, and they told me this was a controversial case - twenty-five authors which I had referenced did not think there was any controversy surrounding these issues! I was told to be quiet and wait. "You really don't want this case to go to court Mr. Stearley." "They would make a big emotional appeal to a jury and would win regardless of what the facts are." Once again, no one was interested in the truth of what had happened.

Another eighteen nervous months dragged by before the settlement was reached. During this time it was revealed to me that the physicians involved had blamed everything on the nurses hoping to shift the burden of any monetary and/or licensure settlements away from themselves. The nurses, on the other hand, had followed the hospital attorney's instructions and remained quiet regarding the physician's mismanagement of the code. The nurses were hung out to dry by this club of physicians - they too were obviously not interested in the truth.

The total amount of the settlement was four million dollars - half to be paid by the institution, and half to be paid by the defendants (there were four physicians and five nurses named in this suit). There were a few other conditions to this settlement which quickly surfaced. The two million paid out by the hospital was immediately to be paid back to the institution - "to pay the patient's bill, of course." The remaining half of the settlement had to be paid by the nine defendants - we were now on our own to come up with two million dollars! Fortunately, I did have malpractice insurance to cover my assigned $70,000 portion. Who determined my portion, or how, was never explained to me, but without this insurance I could have lost my home, all of my personal property, and/or had my wages garnished to eternity!

Yes the hospital attorney serves the hospital, and he had done this well. By settling this case out of court he prevented the institution from receiving any bad publicity, and with all said and done they ended up not having to pay out one red cent. The plaintiff's attorney had done his job well too, and received a high settlement for his client - a client which essentially had no medical or legal basis for receiving any compensation. As for the physicians, their attempts to blame the nurses didn't really help them, but it did show us their true colors. The truth of what had happened was only a side issue from the very beginning of this case.

At least I thought my grief was over, but more bad news arrived in the mail. It seems if you are a health care professional involved in a malpractice litigation your name is permanently recorded in a computer data bank - The National Practitioner Data Bank. This file follows you for life, and employers are strongly encouraged to review this file prior to hiring new employees. Furthermore, what goes into this permanent blemish is the report from your malpractice insurance agent, and the way my agent had painted this picture one would think I was the only defendant and I was accused of being guilty of negligence. Wait one minute! I had not even been taking care of this patient. I had only intervened with the code team to attempt to save this man's life, and now I was listed as being negligent in a permanent employment file! I was given ten days to appeal the report which I did immediately. After four months more of fighting with the insurance agency they agreed to change the wording of their report to reflect how many defendants were involved and to remove the accusation of negligence from the report.

Three years had passed since the beginning of this episode. I had learned how willing to distort the facts the attorneys were, how willing the physicians were to burn the nurses and deny their own errors, how willing the hospital was to push the burden of payment off on to the staff, and how willing the insurance company was to destroy my reputation - and all because I had attempted to perform my job, and assist with the efforts to resuscitate this patient. I could have walked away, not offered any assistance, and never been named in this suit - is this what the powers that be wish to teach the health care community?

The final insult came two months later when I received a registered letter from the State Board of Nursing. It seems they too must review these cases, and they wanted me to know that out of the goodness of their hearts they had decided not to revoke my nursing license! This was the last straw. I have since become very legally conscious, have consulted with several attorneys, and have spent time in the library reviewing case law on nursing issues. I will never allow myself to be put in that position again! I have also prepared some suggestions for all nurses so all of us can practice Defensive Nursing...

Chart Defensively

Throughout our careers we are taught not to do any "negative charting". This is charting which might implicate negligence or poor practice from another health care provider. Somehow the implication is that it is our responsibility to mask the truth - to lie, to cover-up what has really taken place. I say chart the truth and let the dust settle where it will. Notify physicians of everything and chart their names clearly. I can guarantee you once involved in a legal battle they will happily burn you to save their own skin.

If there is a call list of physicians to consult, be assertive and go to the top when your patient's needs are not being met by those lower in command - chart it all. Don't just chart what has been done, chart any suggestions you might have given as well. At least the record will demonstrate you were pursuing your patient's interests. I can't tell you how many times I received immediate attention when I ended a conversation with a doctor by saying the words, "Ok, I will chart accordingly."

Notify your manager, in writing, of any patient situation which did not receive appropriate attention from the physicians. Also send a letter any time you feel staffing is inadequate or your staff is under-skilled to meet your patient's needs. The paper trail you create today will build credibility for managing future problems. One of the first questions directed to me during my deposition was whether or not I felt staffing was adequate. This question was followed by, "Did you ever notify your manager of potential staffing problems?" And, "Where is your written memorandum to support what you're saying?" Don't assume for a moment that addressing such issues verbally with you manager is adequate. An attorney will always ask for written documentation, or else "you must not have done what you claim."

Learn about what legal charting is, and is not. Each of the five hospitals which I have worked for had their own system of charting. Some used more than one system, and most would not cover you legally. Computer charting, for example, only allows you so much space, and so many descriptions of your care to chart. If you write on a computer printout, or chart nurses notes separately, you can be accused of tampering with a legal document and falsifying the record. The nurse providing care for the patient in my lawsuit was accused of just that. Computer charting hurt us in another issue. Because the nurse had signed out a narcotic on the narcotics record, administered it to the patient, and then recorded it on the computer, the two times recorded showed an eight minute difference - we were then accused of giving two doses of the medication when in fact only one had been given.

"Charting by exception" is the new twist which management has tried to sell us. What this means is you have protocols or standards of care which you initial. These protocols can cover simple procedures such as the insertion of a foley catheter, or complex protocols such as with advanced cardiac life support (ACLS). The selling point is you will no longer have to chart all of the meticulous details which you perform - you simply initial the list. While this may increase nurses' autonomy in a small way, and possibly save some time, the problem inherent with this system is protocols can become so numerous, and have so many steps listed, if you fail to perform even just one step of an initiated protocol then not only are you guilty of failing to meet this newly defined standard of practice, but having initialed it you have also falsified the patient's permanent legal record.

Hospitals are also trying to use protocols to absolve themselves of the legal concept of "respondent superior" which states the institution is responsible for the actions of its employees. By initialing a protocol, you could be taking responsibility off of their shoulders and placing it squarely on yours. One legal expert I consulted informed me that simply because a protocol existed at my institution I would be obligated to follow it - whether I initialed it or not!

Traditionally, no written standards of practice existed. In court, the standard has been determined by comparing your actions with those of what a prudent nurse would do in the same or similar set of circumstances. Hospital administrators are now jumping at the opportunity to define standards of practice to shift the burden of responsibility to the bedside nurse. If you think you can use staffing shortages as a defense for not meeting standards formulated in these protocols, think again. Unless you created that paper trail I mentioned earlier throughout the institution's administration you will have nothing to support your claims.

It appears narrative charting remains the best in terms of documenting what care has performed without compromising nurses legally.

Maintain Your Own Personnel File

Last year I discovered my institution maintains two separate personnel files on all of its employees. One is kept in the personnel office and serves as a business record of your employment. The other is kept by the manager and contains evaluations and whatever else has been deemed fit to be placed there. (I have even observed copies of my published articles, such as this one, placed in this file when she has pulled it out to discuss some issue of my employment.) I am only allowed access to my business file. I am not allowed to place any positive records of my achievements or performance in the manager's file. I can place these documents in my business file, but I was assured by my manager whenever I terminated my employment at this institution these additions would be burned. Only the basic facts of my employment dates and wages would be maintained from this file.

The important file which concerns my performance is top secret, and is for their use only. (I was told this is a common business practice.) Consequently, the only way I can be sure I am fairly represented is to maintain my own file. I have copies of every evaluation, every letter of appreciation from a patient or a staff member, every continuing education unit earned, every class or inservice I have taught, every committee served on -basically everything which has advanced myself professionally in any way. This file has disarmed my manager's negative accusations on more than one occasion.

Maintain a Professional Journal

Virtually anything can, and should, be recorded in a personal work journal. My journal has helped me to recall specific patient events, specific conversations with managers, and many seemingly not so important details which have later assisted me in dealing with false accusations leveled at me by some of the administrative staff. I have eliminated many wasted hours of discussion by being able to pull out my journal and state the exact date, time, place, words spoken, and outcomes surrounding many situations.

At one institution I was able to use my journal to convince the personnel department my managers were harassing me regarding some editorials I had published in the local newspaper. Simply producing a document listing dates, times, and events sent shivers through the personnel representative when I discussed whether or not I needed to file a grievance. Later, when I consulted an attorney about this situation I was complemented repeatedly for having maintained such accurate records. This employment journal should not contain elements about your personal life as it may someday be subpoenaed for court, and most of us do not want our personal lives on public display.

I have also found that keeping a journal is a very good stress reduction tool. It allows me to reflect on events, learn more about myself as a person, and move on - clearing my mind. As a writer, a journal is a must - just think of all of the good stories waiting to be written lying on those pages.

Learn About Your Rights As An Employee

Understanding some basics about labor law is a necessity in the turbulent atmosphere of health care reform. Become familiar with legal newsletters. One of the best I located in our library is "The Regan Report on Nursing Law." This newsletter presents brief synopses of case law concerning any issue which you hopefully will not find yourself facing someday.

There are also legal cases presented in some nursing journals such as in Revolution's "War Stories." Read these and learn from your colleagues experiences.

There are many legal organizations waiting to assist you with your questions. Make yourself a phone list and include numbers for the local offices of: the Occupational Safety and Health Administration (OSHA), the National Employment Lawyers Association (NELA), the U.S. Department of Labor - including the Division of Wage and Hour, the National Labor Relations Board (NRLB), and the Equal Employment Opportunity Commission (EEOC).

Hire Your Own Attorney

If at all possible, when faced with a legal situation, hire your own attorney. This individual will be there to represent you - not a hospital, and not an insurance company. You need to have your own interests represented.

Build Supportive Relationships With Your Co-Workers

Nurses must learn to be supportive of each other. I have seen many situations in which staff nurses have been so willing to back-bite one another that they have undermined their own common causes. I have also witnessed times when nurses have united, marched into their manager's office en masse, and walked out with satisfaction in hand. Nurses have always been effective communicators when advocating their patients - it is time to advocate ourselves!

If we are truly to advance professionally, then we must unite and support each other.Remember, you own your license, not your employer. You decide your career's direction, And you are the best person to defend yourself in a crisis. Defensive nursing can promote a more secure working environment, and help prevent the exploitation of all nurses.

- This last issue of professional support, or lack there of, is perhaps no better illustrated than in the profession of nursing. Back-biting and in-fighting seem to be the rule. The next chapter illustrates how this is a no-win situation for nurses.

*****

Chapter 20

Professional Jealousy - The No Win Factor
*Published in **REVOLUTION** - The Journal of Nurse Empowerment*
Volume 4, Number 4, Pages 52-53.

I had just received the news of my latest nursing research project having been accepted for publication. I had spent some 200 hours of my own personal time designing research tools, collecting the data, analyzing this data, preparing the manuscript, and submitting it to various journals. All of the hard work was now earning its reward. I wasn't even receiving an honorarium or payment, but I was ecstatic! The article highly profiled the institution where I was employed - at that time - so I felt I would be in good standing with my management. The first words of congratulations arrived, and I was psyched up for my next project.

This honeymoon phase was short-lived, however, and the tone of the comments quickly changed. One staff member approached me and said, "I see that you were published." "You sure milked this program for all it's worth." One of clinical specialists made a point of tracking me down to inform me, "You really need to have a masters degree to be considered credible when publishing nursing research." And, during a staff meeting, in front of my peers, an assistant manager down played my research by stating, "Oh, you were just writing that article to get paid for it."

My own manager, who I thought would be thrilled, told me that I had better let her review anything which I wrote in the future because, after all, she had a Ph.D., and it was she who knew how to do research.

After submitting my plans for a second research project, my manager told me, "You're beating a dead horse." "You need to find something else to do." Yet another manager called me into her office to inform me, "You have demonstrated an entrepreneurial spirit, and now you need to stop this and come back to work within our system."

A third manager was a bit more blunt. "No one is interested in what you have to say." And, as if these comments were not enough, another manager let me know that I was perceived as some sort of "threat to authority", and added, "You are articulate; therefore you are dangerous because someone might actually believe something you say."

What is going on here? I thought nurses should support one another and work together to advance our profession. Where did all of this petty competitiveness and animosity come from? I can only hope that what I experienced is the exception and not the rule, or else we will always have trouble uniting to face the challenges confronting nursing.

There is no need to seek out a definition of jealousy from Webster's Dictionary. We all know what this behavior encompasses, and we are all familiar with its destructive effects. What is important is why this behavior is so prevalent in nursing, why its so detrimental, and how it can be avoided.

Not so ironically, I found the majority of literature concerning jealous behavior under the heading of Child Psychology. Of course, one must admit jealousy is a rather childish behavior, but this dysfunctional behavior may very well be at the heart of many problems which adult nurses have when dealing with each other on a daily basis.

Low self-esteem and competitiveness seem to be requirements to join the ranks of nursing. The real problems develop when this pattern of behavior takes on a pathological significance. Constant discontent with oneself is not only pervasive in nursing, but it is enslaving, contaminating every relationship and making each attempt at communication an arena for competition.

Why is self-esteem such a problem for nurses? Generally speaking, nurses are socialized to be subservient. In the traditionally paternalistic, male-dominated fields of medicine and management, the female-dominated field of nursing routinely takes orders and learns very quickly that it is somehow wrong to question those orders.

Nurses are high achievers, educated with the expectation of accomplishing idealistic clinical goals. All of us have experienced some form of "reality shock" as we made our transition from student to practicing nurse, and most of us have devalued ourselves if we failed to live up to our ideals.

It's bad enough we do this to ourselves, but our managers fuel more failure by continually demanding we do more with less so they can toe the bottom line. Again, we fail to deliver the ideal care we were taught our patients deserve, and we blame ourselves.

There is a pervasive message that management does not care about bedside nurses, as we are rarely acknowledged or praised, but rewarded with only greater expectations. We carry a heavy burden of responsibility to our clients, our employers, and our physicians. What nurse could succeed in such an environment -an environment geared for failure? And if managers do not support the front line care givers, and create a practice arena geared for failure, then they must not value the patients we are trained to serve. An extremely negative attitude to impart to those of us at the bedside.

Too often, nurses internalize these negative feelings, losing their ability to empower themselves, either individually or collectively. When people feel badly about themselves, or their circumstances, it is difficult to feel good about anyone else's good fortune.

The ensuing competitive behavior is further aggravated by other circumstances. For all of the expectations to perform, to pursue advanced degrees, to achieve certification in our areas of expertise, we receive limited - if any - rewards.

Promotions for nurses are so few, it makes me wonder what we are competing for? Nurses find themselves competing for recognition, respect, and unofficial power. In nursing, competition, which normally drives systems and individuals to excellence, creates few winners and many losers.

Competition, instead of cooperation, is instilled in nursing neophytes during their academic training. We are taught not only to compete for grades, but to compete to be more "professional." Associate degree students are drilled on how superior their clinical training will be, while bachelor-prepared students are told that only they will be considered to be "professional" nurses. Nursing educators seem to focus more on judging students than truly assisting them to learn and grow. Whether they realize it or not, our academic leaders encourage more infighting! And, with no clear guidelines from our nursing leaders in our professional associations, division remains the rule.

Competition has also become one of the chosen weapons of nurse administrators. Every institution where I have worked has fostered division within the nursing staff. By keeping nurses divided between units and shifts; new-hires and experienced staff; associate, diploma, and bachelor credentials; and favorites and outcasts, managers create an impotent, fractionated workforce.

Deliberate understaffing, a favorite approach to reduce hospital costs, creates more division as nurses judge each other's ability to "cut the mustard" under these extreme working conditions. Face it, the administration has less to worry about from infighting and backbiting than it does from a united staff demanding an improved patient care environment. How can we attain proper nurse-patient ratios, equitable salaries, and decent benefits if we are busy fighting each other?

Faced with such impotence, our self-esteem once again plummets, and we become envious of the few receiving those limited rewards, feeding back into this dysfunctional cycle. Unfortunately, the potential for competition among nurses will probably escalate as projected budgetary constraints result in nursing layoffs.

So what do we do? We are supposed to be professionals, yet we spend more time undermining each other than advancing as a cohesive group. First, I think we need to take our blinders off. The time for denial has passed. We must recognize that, as a group, nurses are more united by a desire to destroy each other than to support each other.

We cannot proceed without identifying our common goals, and we must start by acknowledging that we do have common goals. We must identify those goals and concentrate on ways to cooperate in order to achieve them. Remember, nurses are high achievers and can achieve great things if they chose to do so.

Next we need to recognize each other for our accomplishments, and quit judging and comparing ourselves. We each have unique talents and strengths, and, in the grand scheme of things, we all have equal significance. Supportive relationships not only bring us closer together, but research shows that job stress decreases as cooperative efforts increase.

Finally, we must recognize our enemies and take unified action to address our grievances. We are already exposed to life-threatening diseases, mechanical and electrical hazards, radiation, chemicals, drugs, combative patients, poor management, long hours, short staffing, sexual stereotyping -you name it! Must we fight each other too!

For nurses, infighting is clearly a no-win situation. As healthcare changes in this country, we better be prepared to stand side by side to face the challenges before us.

Post-Script

With the dysfunctional behavior which runs so rampant in our profession, one must ask if our so-called nursing leaders have been infected with the same disease. The answer, I believe, is a resounding YES!

The next chapter illustrates just what happens when your professional association gets involved with policy making. Policy making which they tell us is supposed to advance our profession. Policy making which is controlled by nursing administrators and nursing academia. Policies determined, once again, by individuals who have not been near a sick patient for so long that they have forgotten what it takes to care for that person. Weak-willed policies which sell nurses out. And they call this leadership?

*****

Chapter 21

Restructuring and the ANA - Who's Side Are They On?
Published in **REVOLUTION - The Journal of Nurse Empowerment**
Fall 1994, Volume 4, Number 3, Pages 36-42.

The major buzz words in hospital management circles these days are "restructuring" and "redesign". "Downsizing", "layoffs", "being let go", "pink slips" - the words keep changing to accommodate the politically correct world of double speak, but the realities are still the same - "don't let the door hit your behind on the way out."

Believe me, I know the fallout of restructuring all too well as my position was just eliminated. After eight years of loyal job performance, and five research studies demonstrating the cost effectiveness of my program, I was told, "Good luck." I am but one of the many nurses being terminated across this country, all of us flattened and demoralized by the budget steamroller.

Nurses are beginning to ask hard questions, "What will happen to our patients?" "What are the forces driving these massive changes in healthcare?" "Where are our nursing leaders in the American Nurses Association (ANA), the so-called "voices" of the American Nurse, and where does our national organization stand on these critical issues?"

Some history, I believe, must precede any answers to these questions. In the late 1980s, a nationwide trend spread throughout the business sector to cut costs and streamline bureaucracy. Major companies, such as General Motors (GM) and International Business Machines (IBM) began reducing their work forces. Hospital administrators, recognizing there was more profit to be made, joined in the "downsizing party." Predominately, the general business sector targeted middle management for their reductions - not front line personnel as has become the case in the nursing profession.

Ironically, the major reason cited in the literature for restructuring patient care is the present nursing shortage. This shortage, while hidden by reducing FTEs and imposing mandatory overtime for the staff remaining, is projected to increase as the demand for professional nursing care continues to grow. All of the sources I researched cited a greater need for RNs, so why did my manager tell me there was a glut of nurses and that we were all expendable.

If there is a shortage of skilled nursing care, why have thousands of nurses been laid off across the nation? And why are thousands more in peril of having their positions eliminated?

It appears the encroaching utilization of "unlicensed assistive personnel" (UAP), or registered care technicians, or technical clinical associates - all euphemisms for minimally trained healthcare providers designed to supplement care provided by RNs - is the answer.

These unlicensed, unskilled, minimally trained assistants are now being used to replace RNs instead of supplementing their care as originally intended. Unconcerned with the shortage of skilled care, it appears nursing administrators are aggravating this shortage as they are more concerned with cutting their budgets to preserve their own inflated salaries! (One director of nursing in my town makes more money than the Governor of the state!)

Another rationale for restructuring is a change in the prospective payment system. Fees are capitated based on diagnosis in attempt to eliminate unnecessary treatments. Thus, the less expense incurred to treat a patient the greater percentage of the capitated fee is profit. The advent of these diagnosis-related groups (DRGs) has resulted in hospitals receiving sicker patients whose illnesses are treated so quickly their hospital stay demands the highest skilled care available. This increase in patient acuity inevitably increases the demand for highly skilled nurses. Management's desire to lower costs and increase profits by replacing professional nurses with UAP will ultimately result in higher patient morbidity and mortality. It is faulty logic to conclude that as third party reimbursement for services decreases, patient safety becomes secondary to profit margins.

Quality of care issues have resulted in the creation of a one-billion-dollar per year quality oversight business composed of professional review organizations, the Joint Commission on Accreditation of Hospitals Organization, state and local health department reviews, and institutional quality assurance programs.

Consumers have also pushed for better care as our society is beginning to become more health conscious and more knowledgeable about what good health care is and isn't. Quality issues, including emergency interventions, medication errors, patient falls, and noscomial infections, are directly related to the number of skilled R.N.s staffed. Its a simple correlation: the greater the number of R.N.s, the greater the quality of care.

Again we are left to wonder why restructuring is leading to the elimination and replacement or R.N.s when it appears just the opposite is required to protect and promote the health of all Americans. So just where is this redesign in healthcare going?

Recently, many nursing administrators have attempted to apply product line management theory to the skilled delivery of patient care. The "product" in this framework is the patient, and the caregivers are merely components on the healthcare assembly line. Nurses are losing their identity as they become labeled "the maternal-child product line", "the emergency-trauma product line", and the "medical-surgical product line."

It is now very convenient for nurse-managers to shift newly classified "nurse resources" to various units under these broad classifications - this used to be called floating. Nurses no longer have names or faces. We have become interchangeable parts in the assembly line of managed healthcare. This type of impersonal management style reduces the compassionate delivery of care to the same level as the mass production of coat hangers - "cheaper is better" and "quantity versus quality."

In my observation and experience, hospital administrators view nurses as nothing more than labor - labor which is costly and serves only to minimize the institution's profits. So crunch the numbers and to heck with quality! After all, lower quality care translates to expensive and profitable patient complications. As a friend of mine in business school told me, "Nothing personal, it's just business."

Quality has become a secondary issue to most administrators, although there is no shortage of politically correct rhetoric that attempts to convince the public that, much as the 16th century physicians believed, bleeding the patient is somehow therapeutic.

So what are the proposals for restructuring the delivery of nursing care? The types of programs are as numerous as there are hospitals, but clearly they are not empowering for RNs.

The "Patient Centered Framework," originating from the District of Columbia General Hospital, is one of the more favorable alternatives for restructuring nursing care delivery. This system recognizes and promotes the quality of services with commitment to integrating care surrounding the patient's needs. The institution's primary focus would be its support and care of its primary care providers. What a novel idea! Also, it is believed the costs would be minimal, compared to the long-range health and viability of the institution.

In this scheme, collaboration would be the rule among all components of healthcare delivery, the management structure being represented by an inverse pyramid where the patients make up the largest base, followed by direct caregivers, and with management occupying the smallest component or point of the pyramid.

Initial evaluation of this framework showed a lowering of RN turnover from 33 percent to 19 percent; a decrease in length of stay for the patient by one to four days; a 55 percent improvement in discharge planning; a 57 percent increase in quality assurance data; a 57 percent increase in patient teaching; and a 7% increase in individual plans of care.

Finally, there was a significant reduction in patient re-admissions - in Ob-Gyn alone, the re-admission rate dropped from 40 percent to one percent. In short, this plan demonstrated that an increase in the number of R.N.s at the bedside, along with an increase in support personnel, decreased patient mortality and morbidity significantly.

It is important to note that not all forms of the Patient-Centered Care are applied in the same manner from institution to institution. In fact, some administrators have chosen to bastardize this approach, and instead of increasing the number of R.N.s and providing more support personnel, they have chosen to replace R.N.s with more UAP. Having more unskilled, minimally trained workers hanging around does little to improve the quality of care, and while R.N.s may be completing paperwork, i.e. care plans, this does not translate to improved care either. As with all great human ideas, there are more humans waiting to take such an idea, distort it to make a profit, and claim they are serving their fellow man. (For more specific information on how such a good idea can go wrong refer back to the chapter entitled Patient-Focused Care - The End To Hospital Nursing?)

The majority of other plans for redesign are not as favorable to R.N.s as was the original design by D. C. General Hospital. Their proponents attempt to slant their presentation to make it appear that lowering numbers of professional staff directing unlicensed assistive personnel will somehow magically translate into a more professional role for the R.N. - patient care issues aside. The Pro-ACT model from New Brunswick, New Jersey, is one such example.

Beginning with the cliché that "times of crisis and great change are also times of great opportunity," the authors of Pro-ACT assert that creating a triad system of R.N. Clinical Care Managers, R.N. Primary Nurses, Licensed Practical Nurses (L.P.N.s), and UAP will result in improved job satisfaction, improved patient satisfaction, cost reduction, and improvement in the quality of patient care.

These are high-falutin' claims, considering their data is marginal and fluctuating. The authors of ProACT claim that, under their plan, normal shifts in patient acuity occurred; patient satisfaction with direct nursing care remained unchanged; patient satisfaction with housekeeping or nursing support services increased; and nursing staff satisfaction improved initially, but then declined to slightly above baseline. Subjective quality-of-care measures such as patient compliance and outcome showed modest increases, while objective measures such as incidents and infections remained unchanged.

In the ProACT plan costs of nursing care from using UAP versus R.N.s decreased, and individual patient costs decreased marginally when they were related to early discharge. Overall, hospital profits increased slightly when there was an increase in the volume of patients and beds were speedily emptied to make room for the next patient. All of their data were marginal, except that patients received better housekeeping - and we know how important image versus real quality is. In fact, the slight increase in hospital profits was achieved by dumping R.N.s and dumping patients.

We also know early discharge can compromise patient safety. This addresses another aspect of restructuring - transferring patients to the next healthcare delivery system. It is now common practice to regard primary, secondary, and even tertiary healthcare, as part of the "community system," a philosophy which dictates that a hospitalized patient be "dumped" as soon as possible to a nursing home or to his or her own home. Early discharge shifts the costs away from the hospital. This, as I have mentioned, is now called collaboration - sharing the patient's illness to maximize all available reimbursement.

While the ProACT model serves to illustrate a slightly better application of the use of UAP, thus still retaining some licensed individuals, by far the major emphasis for restructuring concerns the high usage of UAP and a monumental reduction in the R.N. workforce.

Several types of UAP models have been proposed, including: a return to traditional team nursing which uses very low numbers of professional staff to direct large numbers of workers who usually receive on-the-job training; a modified version of team nursing employing "super aides" who have received eight weeks of training; the "unit assistant" model which incorporates the roles of clerk and nursing assistant; and the technician model which trains aides to provide advanced care such as IV therapy, assistance with invasive procedures, and the monitoring of invasive lines.

These models pose yet another irony. Although one of the major arguments for employing UAP is to relieve the R.N. from doing nonprofessional housekeeping details which are distracting her or him from patient care, in reality, nursing administrators are training UAP to perform skilled nursing tasks and, in essence, setting up a system in which UAP substitute for R.N.s.

So where does the American Nurses Association, our representative political body, stand on these issues? In order to answer this question, I decided to attend the A.N.A.'s National Convention in San Antonio, Texas, last June 10-15. The word "shocked" would be an understatement to describe what I observed at this giant "pep rally."

I am glad the A.N.A is described as an association versus an organization, because organized they were not! The first day consisted of registration and exclusive meeting for the various delegates. Registration for us peon R.N.s consisted of a two hour wait in line, as individuals struggled and failed to electronically document our payment and course selections. Course material was determined by title listings only. Later, I discovered the titles were often not the slightest bit reflective of the course content.

The official opening of the convention came on Saturday, June 11th, with an appearance by Hillary Clinton! After wading through the security teams, guard dogs, and A.N.A. staff, I found myself perched near the top of the arena listening endlessly to Fleetwood Mac's "Rumors." It was showtime as Virginia Trotter Betts, the A.N.A.'s president, walked into the auditorium side-by-side with Hillary Clinton.

After Ms. Betts repeated the A.N.A.'s pledge to back the Clinton healthcare reform package - managed healthcare - the First Lady presented an articulate speech. But, it appeared to me that most of what she said was falling on the wrong ears.

Mrs. Clinton referred to the fact that nurses "care more about need than greed," and stated that 27 percent of all U.S. hospitals were down-sizing and eliminating nurses, which was not representative of true healthcare reform. While she offered no specific solutions to the problems she highlighted, she certainly made an eloquent presentation. The problem, however, was the First Lady was speaking primarily to an audience composed of the very administrators who are laying off R.N.s, and to complacent A.N.A. delegates and administrative staff members -

deaf ears to say the least!

One of my favorite moments of this conference came when the exhibition hall opened on Sunday, June 12th. Nurses, it seems, are so frequently rewarded for their efforts with meaningless trinkets that they have come to accept them as an important form of recognition. As I walked through the hall to view the exhibits, I was literally knocked out of the way as an A.N.A delegate literally dove into a booth to secure a handful of give-away ink pins.

One time, I was hit so hard that I was knocked against another person and almost fell to the floor. This, I thought is power in motion. If only A.N.A. delegates fought as hard for the plight of staff nurses as they did for these trinkets, we would have the most powerful lobby movement in this country!

After three days of sessions, I managed to stumble into two important seminars concerning the use of assistive personnel. To my chagrin, however, I learned that the A.N.A. representatives were unwilling to discuss the Association's official policy statement regarding the use of UAP. My comments and questions were continually redirected to the issue of R.N.s learning how to properly delegate tasks to UAP, the better to avoid liability for inadequate care.

In this regard, nurses were encouraged to document incidents and purchase an A.N.A. publication entitled, "Registered Professional Nurse and Unlicensed Assistive Personnel." The A.N.A.'s attorney, Winifred Y. Carson, J.D., seemed to be presenting this issue with great urgency, stressing the legal vulnerability which R.N.s now faced.

During this same session, Peggy K. Jones, M.S.N., M.B.A., the Vice-President of Patient Care Services at St. Francis Medical Center in Trenton, New Jersey, began her lecture with a disclaimer that she was not, in any way, a representative of the A.N.A. and that her opinions were not necessarily the same as the A.N.A.'s. Ms. Jones attacked the use of UAP and cited several research studies showing that the higher the percentage of R.N.s on the staff, the lower the patient mortality and morbidity statistics. She said that R.N.s were needed at the bedside to promote optimum patient outcome!

Her lecture ended with an overwhelming majority of attendees asking how to implement the use of UAP in their individual practice settings and asking for the A.N.A guidelines to assist them in cutting down their R.N. workforce. Only two questions were asked about quality and practice issues!

I decided to pursue the A.N.A.'s policy statement. One staff member informed me she had no idea of how I could get a copy, while another told me I could not obtain one. I proceeded to the A.N.A. representative's booth and found a more helpful person who told me that the A.N.A. no longer distributed policy statements - not even to its members! I learned I could obtain a copy only if I purchased the A.N.A. publication about the use of UAP. So I purchased this booklet at the cost of $6.95, plus tax. Now that's representation!

As a member of the national association which is supposed to represent R.N.s, I was only entitled to see their official policy statement concerning my profession by buying it! Hillary Clinton's words echoed in my ears - this group of nurses cared "more about need than greed!"

What I discovered in the A.N.A.'s publication, "Registered Professional Nurses and Unlicensed Assistive Personnel," were two position statements and one attachment. The first policy statement was entitled, "Registered Nurse Education Relating To The Utilization of Unlicensed Assistive Personnel," and was dated April 13, 1992. The second policy statement was entitled, "Registered Nurse Utilization of Unlicensed Assistive Personnel," dated December 11, 1992. The attachment was entitled "Definitions Related to A.N.A. 1992 Positions Statements On Unlicensed Assistive Personnel."

So what is the A.N.A.'s position regarding these issues? Well, it was easy to see why they didn't want to discuss them at their conference! Immediately, the dates disturbed me since these issues had been around for some time and massive changes have taken place in the American healthcare system over the past two years. Besides, neither I nor any of my colleagues were aware of these policies existence. But, their content was the real shocker.

Basically, the A.N.A. determined that UAP are here now, are here to stay, and will increase in number. Consequently, their policy was an attempt to contrive some standards of practice for the use of UAP and to state that R.N.s are in charge of them.

To me, this is a sell-out - a policy of aquiescence. Instead of fighting for their supposed constituency - the R.N.s who staff our nation's hospitals - buy opposing the use of UAP, the A.N.A.'s policy accepts our fate, steps aside, and warns us that R.N.s will be liable for the actions of our unskilled replacements!

The A.N.A.'s position statements do not support the professional registered nurses they are supposed to represent, and they seem to support the move to mothball us. Is the A.N.A. trying to give our profession away?

Today, as R.N.s are beginning to delegate patient care to UAP, where do we stand? Not on very solid ground! Not only will we be held liable for any wrongful acts committed by UAP, but we have just taken a hit from the U.S. Supreme Court. In brief, when nurses working in an Ohio nursing home complained to their manager about poor working conditions, they were "rewarded" with termination. Seeking protection granted under the National Labor Relations Act (NLRA) an Administrative Law Judge ruled in their favor and ordered their reinstatement. However, the nursing home managers appealed, and the Sixth Circuit Court stated that since the nurses were directing UAP, they were to be classified as supervisors, nor employees, and therefore had no protections under the NLRA.

The U.S. Supreme Court upheld this ruling when the National Labor Relations Board Appeal the Circuit Court ruling, and now it appears all of us who direct L.P.N.s, nurse assistants, or even unit secretaries, will be classified as supervisors, and will have lost all protection under federal labor law.

The A.N.A. states it is "deeply disturbed" by the May 23, 1994 ruling. It sure is comforting to know the Association which is too weak to come out in support of R.N.s and against the use of UAP is "disturbed." While the various administrators of the A.N.A. sit insulated in their offices, it will be the R.N.s on the front-lines who are being replaced by UAP. Thank you for your support!

The Tri-council for Nursing, composed of the American Association of Colleges of Nursing, The American Nurses Association, the American Organization of Nurse Executives, and the National League for Nurses, has issued a statement accepting the use of UAP as directed by R.N.s . They state: "The ultimate aim is to reallocate nursing and non-nursing activities to enable the registered nurse to focus on the patient." Come on now! Anyone who has worked in a team-nursing system can tell you the use of UAP serves only one purpose - to reduce institutional costs.

As a former nursing assistant and present R.N., I can tell you first hand that team nursing keeps the R.N. away from the patient and greatly diminishes the quality of care. Lofty statements from administrators, who have nothing but profit and protecting their own inflated salaries in mind, do little to help bedside nurses and their unsuspecting patients.

Are there other ways the A.N.A. will dis-empower the R.N.s they are supposed to be representing? Well, on Monday, June 13, 1994, during the national convention, the A.N.A.'s House of Delegates voted the A.N.A. should show its support for staff nurses by articulating a vision statement designed to "ensure nurses are essential providers in all practice settings in a restructured healthcare system."

I don't know how this "statement" is going to ensure anything for R.N.s except the loss of collective bargaining power. I may be wrong, but I believe labor law is very specific about groups of employees being classified as providing "essential services." If this classification is made, just as it was in 1980 during the air traffic controllers' strike, nurses will be ordered back to work or face immediate termination if they strike. While there is no question about the value of nursing services, I think nurses might want to phrase their "vision statements" with a little more "vision" with regard to how they may undermine their own power.

When you really think about it, making a statement about R.N.'s value in the workforce is pretty lame. It does nothing to truly support us, nor does it protect or save nursing positions. In fact, when it comes to making statements, the A.N.A. has shown it has no backbone at all - they can't even draft a position statement opposing the use of UAP as replacements for registered nurses! Just who's side are they on?

On Saturday, June 18, 1994, after the conference was over, I received a call from a representative of the A.N.A. who was seeking donations to support the association's political action agenda. As she asked me for a contribution of $100, I wondered exactly what "action" she had in mind. When I told her I had been laid off and was, as a result of restructuring at my former institution, currently unemployed, she replied, "Well Mr. Stearley, there is as hospital on every street corner, I'm sure you won't have any trouble finding a job, so could you at least send us ten dollars?"

I guess she didn't understand that hospitals on every street corner are laying off R.N.s and hiring UAP. Her concern for my situation, and all other R.N.s facing this crisis, was "underwhelming."

◆ As a reminder as to how important having R.N.s at the bedside, I offer you the next chapter. While the ANA gives lip service to defending the role of the RN, they manufacture policies which cut our legs out from under us. If not convinced yet as to how important it is to have professionals skilled in the art of patient assessment than consider some of the risks you will face upon entering the hospital......

*****

Chapter 22

True Lies, True Risks

In the past few months a number of hospital horror stories have managed to land on the front pages of newspapers around the country. I hear stunned people in supermarkets talking about the man in Florida who had the wrong leg amputated. I listen to radio announcers aghast that a woman undergoing a mastectomy in Michigan had the wrong breast removed. A renowned Boston health care journalist goes to one of the most prestigious cancer hospitals in the country only to have her insides fried with four times the appropriate dosage of the chemotherapeutic agent - she died an agonizing death. The wrong man disconnected from his ventilator suffocates. A 5 year old child receives chemotherapy for four days instead of seizure medication and may be unable to have her own children, presuming she lives to child bearing age.... These tales not only send shivers up our spines, but it makes us ask, just what is going on?

Well, we all have good reason to question the care being delivered in our medical institutions. The debate on health care reform has finally sparked some examination of this massive bureaucracy. In fact, up to now, the system has practiced medicine on us with impunity, and some would say "practice" is the operative word in this statement. While there are many kind hearted and well-meaning individuals in the medical community, what kind of quality control can truly exist in a system where you can justify absolutely anything by stating, "We were only trying to help?"

If you have ever signed on for a medical treatment you will most probably hear one number quoted to you - two-percent. Almost every procedure, test, or surgery is described as having a two-percent risk. What about adjustments to take into account different patient histories, skill of the physician, or variations in practice settings? No, usually procedures are presented as carrying a 2% risk of bleeding, infection, stroke, heart attack, or death, but current studies seem to indicate your risks are much higher. Not only the ones traditionally discussed with you at the bedside as you sign the consent form, but other conveniently unmentioned risks.

The 1991 Harvard University Study of New York Hospitals indicated 3.7% of all inpatients suffered from the traditionally quoted risks - bleeding, infection, stroke, heart attack, or death. This same study revealed you have a 1% risk of suffering a permanent disability or death related to medical negligence. One-percent doesn't sound too bad until you consider the fact that 4 million patients visit their physicians daily in this country according to the American Medical Association (AMA). That's 40,000 potential negligent injuries daily, and it is estimated that 180,000 patients die each year as a result of physician induced injury. Approximately 20% of these injuries are caused by medication errors with the remaining being caused by medical instrumentation.

As early as 1981, Gertman Steel reported in the New England Journal of Medicine that 36% of hospital patients suffered medically inflicted injuries, of which 25% were serious or life threatening. A classic example of such injury is that of the pneumothorax or collapsed lung. Needle aspiration procedures, draining fluid from the lining of the lungs, and placing large bore catheters for infusions and monitoring generate 54% of all of the collapsed lungs occurring in the hospital setting. These injuries prolong hospital stays, increase cost, and contribute to the fatalities already described.

Many studies have highlighted the incidence and nature of medication errors. In 1991, Dr. S. E. Bedell reported, in the Journal of the American Medical Association, that 64% of all cardiac arrests occurring in hospitals were not only preventable, but were caused by the inappropriate use of prescription medication. In the November 15, 1994 issue of Hospital Practice, Dr. Robert Schrier reports that once hospitalized you have an 18% to 30% chance of experiencing an adverse drug event, and following your physician's orders to take prescription medication results in 60,000 to 140,000 deaths each year.

Physician's instruments and medication errors aside, what about hospital acquired infections? In his book "Managing Hospital Infection Control for Cost Effectiveness", Dr. Robert Haley documents 6% of all in-patients develop hospital acquired infections. These infections account for 20,000 deaths annually, and contribute to an additional 60,000 hospital deaths. Urinary tract infections make up 40% of these noscomial infections, surgical wounds 25%, respiratory infections 15%, bloodstream infections 5%, with the remainder classified as "other". Just lying in a hospital bed predisposes us to a 7% rate of developing a pressure ulcer and another potential wound infection.

What about the possibility of infection from a blood transfusion should we require one? The 1993 Heymann and Brewer study published in the American Journal of Infection Control indicated that while blood transfusion infection rates are relatively low, HIV at .0000065% hepatitis at 2 percent, with 20 million units transfused annually we cause 130 new cases of HIV and 400,000 cases of hepatitis each year with prescribed blood products.

Essentially every medical intervention holds the promise of a side effect creating the need for yet another intervention. It's not very comforting to face these potential risks when one also considers that Consumer Reports documents 20% of all tests, procedures, and surgeries as being totally unnecessary in the first place. To compound our fears, consider the fact that autopsy studies reported in the Journal of Pathology showed physicians misdiagnosed the cause of death in 35 to 40 percent of all of their cases! How can anyone prescribe appropriate treatment without truly knowing what illness is afflicting you? It would seem at times that hospital patients get well in spite of medical treatment, not because of it.

Perhaps not all of us would be so willing to consent to treatment if we knew the "true risks" we faced. It's time consumers began to ask hard questions regarding their medical care, and it's time for the medical community to start answering those questions honestly.

Post-Script

The system of health care delivery is dysfunctional. The managers controlling it have forgotten their mission of providing quality patient care. Infractions of morals, ethics, and law abound. Silence protects the "club." And, it is, after all, a club mentality, and silence is the new definition of loyalty.

If you wish to be a member you must play by the rules. You follow instructions which are not always in the best interest of your patients. You must keep quiet even if things go wrong. Even if people die when they didn't have to.

This is a traumatic working environment. We witness all of our society's negative aspects. Illness, suffering, pain, and death with a dose of greed, avarice, deceit, and exploitation. I can confidently state that working in this environment produces metal illness, and the nurses act as if they are victims of "post-tramatic stress disorder" or "battered women's syndrome." With good reason - they are.....

*****

Chapter 23

Battered But Not Beaten - The Politics of Victimization
*Published in **REVOLUTION** - **The Journal of Nurse Empowerment***
Volume 5, Number 1, pages 63-64.

Recently, there have been volumes of articles describing codependent behavior among nurses. So many, in fact, that critics have begun saying we are overusing the popular terminology of victimization.

For instance, in her article, "Under the Influence: The Myth of Professional Codependency," appearing in Revolution: The Journal of Nurse Empowerment's Spring 1994 issue, author Robin Walter rejected the labeling of nurses as being codependent. She warned that nurses should not identify themselves or their profession as being sick and in need of being rescued. While Ms. Walter made some good points, she failed to offer an alternative explanation for the self-sacrificing behavior which erodes our professional power.

If it's not codependency, then what is it? Why have nurses become entrenched in self-victimizing behavior? How is this behavior perpetuated, and how can we break the cycle to emerge as confident, self-directed professionals?

Let's be frank. Nursing is a field composed of 97 percent women, and even as we face the 21st Century, women are regarded and treated as second-class citizens. I can hear the voices of protest already, but even after considering all of the strides which women have made, they still earn between 59 and 77 percent of what men earn while performing comparable work. This is nothing to brag about.

Who, among the two million nurses in this country - excluding nurses administrators - can honestly say they are paid equitably for their professional talents, and work in an optimal patient-care environment?

Face it, nurses have been victimized! Our talents in caring for others have been exploited. We have been taught to be helpless and we blame ourselves for not being everything to everyone. In reality, we are fault, not for inadequate performance, but for allowing ourselves to be victims.

Call it whatever you want, guilt and self-blame contribute to our lack of self-esteem which, in turn, decrease our ability to stand up for ourselves. Guilt, self-blame, decreased self-esteem, and helplessness - these are the elements in the revolving door which keep nurses spinning in circles.

To break this cycle, we must begin by admitting the cycle exists, by identifying those who exploit it, and by understanding its political significance.

What nurses experience in their places of work mimics "battered women syndrome." It is estimated that over one million women are victims of companion inflicted violence each year. Whether married or single, or whether the abuse is physical or mental, there is no denying this syndrome any longer.

The symptomatology of the battered woman is strikingly similar to the dysfunctional behavior exhibited by nurses: low self-esteem, a sense of worthlessness, isolation, and helplessness. Sound familiar?

One of the most prominent features of this condition is the difficulty women have leaving the source of injury and exploitation. Often, it is the lack of social support and a poor economic situation which traps them in a cycle of abuse: taking it, resolving to leave it, and then returning to it.

From my psychology classes, I remember the concept of "learned helplessness" quite well. Experiments with laboratory animals, such as rats, have shown if you place them in water, and repeated thwart their attempts to swim to safety, they will eventually give up trying and drown.

People, too, often give up their goals after meeting with a certain amount of resistance. And, the resistance which nurses run up against routinely, while trying to secure fair working conditions, is formidable indeed! How many of your colleagues have told you they felt trapped, not by a physical barrier, but by the obstacles to progress which "the system" presents?

It sometimes takes over 20 attempts for a battered woman to leave her abuser before she is successful in not returning to "harm's way." Many women who have broken free say they succeeded only after admitting they were being abused. Maybe it's time for nurses to break free, to surface from denial, and to take back what rightfully is theirs - their own self-respect.

For meaningful changes to take place, nurses have to admit they have been battered, and they must understand who is doing the beating and why. In the traditionally patriarchal healthcare industry, it is easy to see how physicians have put, and kept, nurses "in their place." Nurses are still regarded as "the girls" who are "playing" with life-sized dolls; "the cheerleaders" for doctor heroes (as if all of their own efforts were secondary); and even as the "future homemakers" who will bear the doctors of tomorrow.

While I, as a man, have been subjected to many degrading remarks for becoming a nurse, I have only witnessed the overt sexual harassment which my female counterparts experience. As a male, I can tell you that many male physicians simply regard nurses as eligible girlfriends or mates or a pool of flirtation objects - a pool which is replenished each year by a new graduating class with younger, less experienced "girls" to exploit sexually. What surprises me more, however, is that some women accept this type of treatment without protest. Apparently, they have been socialized to believe sexual exploitation is the norm, and men who are nurturing and supportive are either "abnormal", or to be regarded with suspicion.

Nurses have become better at recognizing and combating physicians' improper behavior by filing complaints and calling "code pinks" when the harassment occurs. But what about our administrators? The type of harassment they inflict on their fellow nurses is more insidious in nature and is compounded by the fact that many of us refuse to believe that "our own" would exploit us.

We know many of our nurse-managers have risen through the ranks of an essentially dysfunctional system, carrying with them the same self-defeating personality traits of the classically abused person. Janet Woititz described this management style -over-critical, over-demanding, demeaning, laissez-faire, and rescuing - which led to her book, The Self-Sabotage Syndrome. This type of leadership style perpetuates the cycle of abuse among nurses, and keeps them "in their place."

In many management journal articles I've read, this "place" is overtly referred to as one occupied by subservient, guilt-motivated, and easily manipulated nurses. It matters not whether this abusive leadership stems from the manager's own neurotic behavior, or is deliberately perpetrated. What matters is the end result - keeping nurses powerless, underpaid, unrecognized, and unsupported. In a word, battered!

The rationale for using such tactics to manage staff nurses is simple: lower costs, higher profits and no hassles from nurses asking to be treated with a little dignity. If this is difficult to believe, I suggest you go to your own nursing library and conduct your own literature review. I was shocked too when I came across titles such as, "Manipulation: Making the Best of It," "Divide and Conquer," "Union Busters," and "Firing Without Fear."

The next logical question, of course, is how do we combat those who batter us?

Again, those who do manage to break the cycle of abuse had to have first admitted they were abused and then recognize the source of their victimization. Nurses must do the same by lifting the veil of deception and seeing who truly supports them. In my experience, hospital nursing managers support hospitals, not nurses.

Proof? I have yet to witness any groups of hospital administrators rush to protest staff nurse layoffs, poor staffing, lack of equipment, dangerous working environments, poor wages, or lack of decent benefits. Under these circumstances, staff nurses must learn to support each other, and stand up against those who attempt to exploit them.

Assertiveness training is a must! We must learn to value and stand up for ourselves. Once we wake up to our own self-worth, we can begin to recognize the worth of all nurses - I have never seen a profession so critical of itself! A profession dedicated to helping others should be proud, not helpless! If we can learn to appreciate ourselves as a group of skilled professionals, we can, as a unified force, demand the administrative support we deserve.

DEMAND !

- We need to demand the proper staffing ratios to provide the care our patients deserve.

- We need to demand the compensation we deserve for our skills.

- We need to demand work environments which provide safety measures, and the equipment necessary, to protect us from the dangers of exposure to toxic chemicals, radiation, electrical hazards, and life-threatening infectious diseases.

- We need to demand an end to the mental abuse inflicted upon us by profit-oriented managers.

- We need to demand that our managers attend good management training courses so they can learn how to value their staff nurses. My father was a career officer in the Air Force, but they didn't just give him command. He was sent to officer's training school. Even the military bureaucracy is more advanced than the nursing bureaucracy. The administrators of the organization trained to kill people are better educated to respect their employees than the administration of the organization dedicated to heal people.

- We need to demand, and keep on demanding, until we are heard! Perhaps the old saying "nice guys finish last" is true. Well, nurses have been "nice guys" long enough. We are tired of being kicked around. It's time for our abusers to learn that we may battered, but we are not beaten!

Post-Script

If you think nurses and patients have been being kicked around just wait till you see what comes of the latest debate on Medicare and Medicaid. These two programs together pay for 20% of all of the health care delivered in this country. Just imagine what will happen in the managed care environment if the proposed cuts are adopted. The current frenzy to eliminate professional registered nurses will escalate! Patient morbidity and mortality will grow exponentially! Corporations will slash and burn healthcare benefits until strict rationing, or denial, of services becomes the rule.

In the next chapter, I take a brief look at the reasoning, or irrationality, behind the move to cut these budgets. Remember, our society is aging. We, ourselves, are aging. Will there be any healthcare for us when we reach 65, or will that become the new cut off point?

Legislators keep up the rhetoric about how their policies will prevent the rationing of care in this country. They tell us we don't want any form of socialized medicine, yet they are all too willing to privatize all medical services and allow economic rationing of health care. Will health care become a rich man's perk?

*****

Chapter 24

Medicare Reform - You Bet Your Life
*Published in the Columbia Missourian
September 25, 1995, page 4A.*

Newt Gingrich, Bob Dole, and the rest of the "Republican Gang" are out to save Medicare. Or are they? Medicare's portion of our nation's 1994's $1 trillion dollar health care tab was almost $200 billion dollars or 20% of the total bill. The question before Congress is will slashing $270 billion dollars from this fund over seven years really accomplish anything more than denying services to an increasing number of elderly citizens?

Focus on short-term gains has plagued this country's economy for many years. Japan's success as an economic giant has largely been credited with their ability to make projections ten years into the future, while American business comparatively looks ten minutes into the future. This short-sighted approach was adopted by our government sometime ago and has resulted in catastrophic short-term debt - debt which we are barely able to pay the interest on, and which cripples our ability to invest more into our society.

Now the politicians in Washington are seeking redemption by wildly slashing and burning anything which could be labeled an "entitlement." This attack appears to be limited, however, when it comes to the politicians themselves who have the best "entitlement" plans in the world including health care and pension funds which dwarf what the average worker could ever expect to earn in his or her lifetime.

Medicare covers hospital and doctor bills for an estimated 32 million Americans. According to the General Accounting Office (GAO), 7 million of these citizens require long-term medical or nursing care. By the year 2000 these numbers will almost double with 62 million Americans receiving benefits and 14 million requiring long-term care.

The groups who rely on Medicare benefits the most are those with fixed incomes, often living in poverty, and often without adequate access to health insurance. Persons over 75 years of age spend 17% of their disposable income on the so-called out-of-pocket health care costs, and those over 85 spend 42% on such costs. As our population ages, it is foolish to believe demand for senior health care is going to diminish or that these costs will somehow decrease.

The Republican plan doesn't take into account the massive changes which are occurring in the composition of our society. There is no accounting for increasing costs related to technology, inflation, or the fraud and profiteering occurring throughout the industry. In fact, the GOP idea of providing vouchers to induce elders to join managed care networks is projected to raise costs instead of lowering them.

Princeton University economist Uwe E. Reinhardt recently examined the numbers and reports the available data is "too crude and confusing to support a hopeful hypothesis." It seems HMOs enjoyed a one-time savings as enrollees were moved out of high-cost plans. This savings is rapidly being erased as premiums for almost all of these managed care plans are rising. Last year's average increase of 9.7% demonstrates the impact increases in technology and an aging society will have on these plans. And, for all the premium dollars collected by HMOs less money was spent on actual health care as their administrative costs eat 31% of their total revenues. Medicare only spends 2% of its contributions on administration allowing the government to channel more into the actual provision of services.

Managed care defeats cost-savings by the very premise which makes it good for the insurance companies which operate it. You spread the cost of illness over all participants - especially the healthy ones who will require little care. To illustrate, the CBO points out 9% of all Medicare recipients are already enrolled in managed care plans, yet these individuals cost the government more than those in traditional fee-for-service plans. How?

The government negotiates a fixed payment per enrollee in HMO plans. The costs of Medicare recipients in a particular region of the country are averaged, and then the government negotiates for a lower fee to try to incur savings. Typically this fee amounts to 95% of the average payment which sounds as though you are saving money, after all, we are paying 5% less of the average cost per individual, right? Well, not exactly. You see the HMO receives this lump sum payment even if the person enrolled requires no health care at all. So when the numbers were actually totaled for those Medicare recipients enrolled in managed care, the CBO discovered it was costing the government 6% more than had it just paid for the services actually rendered. It may sound as though you are paying less for each person, but you are actually paying for services which are never provided.

This is the same reason HMOs do their best to limit services and referrals to specialists - they profit more for the less they provide.

The only way it appears the Republican plan will work is if services are eliminated, beneficiaries are cut, and recipients increase their already high out-of-pocket expenses. It is estimated this proposal will add $1000 annually to each Medicare beneficiary's cost, and where are people living on fixed income expected to raise the money to finance the Republican's scheme?

Essentially the GOP plan would privatize Medicare, and while the American public may very well be resentful of government interference in their lives, they are equally resentful about having their interests turned over to wealthy corporations to be exploited - especially when it involves life and death decisions.

The Republican mantra is that Medicare costs rise 10% each year and this will break the program's budget by the year 2002. The GOP believes it can save Medicare by limiting its growth to 6.4% per year. Ironically, it is well known that Medicare fraud accounts for ten percent of all payments. If the government simply concentrated on eliminating the fraud and abuse of Medicare maybe there would be no need for this debate. Maybe there never has been a need, and for all of the hype the real issue might just be that capital gains tax cut the GOP so desperately wishes to finance for its wealthy supporters.

Post-Script

In the final chapter we must examine "the final chapter" - that is the terminal events of our lives. Unfortunately, more and more of people's final hours are spent strapped into high-tech hospital environments. Impersonal and often painful, the last moments of our lives are where we spend our most health care dollars. And now, it's discovered that total confusion exists with regard to patient's requests as opposed to physician's actions.

Insurance companies, not to be left out, are adding to this confusion by literally buying patient's death benefits through "viatical settlements". And, HMOs seem to wish to turn futile treatment for some into no treatment for all....

*****

Chapter 25

Terminal Chaos
*Published in the Columbia Missourian
January 1, 1996, page 4A.*

When Mr. Winter entered St. Francis-St. George Hospital in Hamilton, Ohio having a massive heart attack, he specifically told his physician not to perform any extraordinary measures to prolong his life. His physician, Dr. Russo, wrote a "DNR" - Do Not Resuscitate - order in his chart. Despite Mr. Winter's personal request, his condition of end-stage heart disease, and the physician's written order, when the crucial moment came Mr. Winter's heart was given an electrical shock and he was successfully resuscitated - or was he? Not only had he suffered the pain and emotional stress of the resuscitation efforts, but he subsequently experienced a paralyzing stroke and died two weeks later in agony leaving a greatly inflated hospital bill behind for his family to pay.

Unfortunately, Mr. Winter's story is becoming all too common in our aging society. As these life and death choices become more necessary, it appears physicians have miles to go before terminal patients can sleep.

A study was launched to evaluate such "wrongful life" cases, and the results were published in the November 22, 1995 issue of the Journal of the American Medical Association (JAMA). Shocking is the only word which can describe the total disregard for patients' wishes reported when it comes to terminal choices. And, if the physicians' desire to heal at all costs is not enough, it appears many of these dying souls were also allowed to suffer with uncontrolled pain prior to their deaths.

The four year study was conducted in two phases examining over 9000 patient cases, and basic communication was identified as a major problem between physicians and their patients. Seventy percent of the time physicians never asked their patients what their preferences were, and only 41% of the study patients were reported to have had any discussions about either their prognosis or cardiopulmonary resuscitation (CPR). Physicians misunderstood their patient's requests 80% of the time regarding CPR, and would only write DNR orders for 50% of the patients requesting them. And, when physicians did write the DNR orders, 46% were written only 2 days before the patient expired. This is long after extraordinary measures had already been inflicted on these terminal patients where common sense could have predicted the final outcome.

The study also confirmed what many of us working in the profession have witnessed, that even if a physician knew a patient's preferences frequently these requests were ignored due to the physician's belief of the patient being uninformed or that the choice not to be resuscitated was not in the best interest of that patient.

Interviews conducted with family members after the patients had died indicated that 50% of all of the conscious patients in the study group had communicated they were experiencing moderate to severe pain during the last three days of their lives. We can only imagine the same percentage of suffering existed in those patients unable to communicate to their loved ones.

Why, with all of the modern technology available to practitioners today, should a patient be denied proper doses of any of a large arsenal of medications available to control a person's suffering? Death may be inevitable for us all, but does it have to be an agonizing one?

Why do physicians ignore the requests of their patients? Well, according to a variety of studies, doctors choosing to over-ride the competent decisions of those they are treating may relate to how these practitioners are socialized and educated.

Physicians are taught that death is not a natural process. Death is a product of disease, and disease is always curable. Wrong. Death is a natural process in total absence of acute, chronic, or debilitating illness, but it has become the enemy of medicine, and the death of a patient has become synonymous with failure of the physician - at least in the physician's mind.

Once these attitudes are imparted it is very difficult to change a physician's practice. Dr. Bernard Lo completed a comprehensive review of clinical studies measuring the reluctance of physicians to change their practice - even in the face of clinical documentation. He discovered that providing physicians information about new drugs, vaccines, and practice guidelines does not alter their practice. "Physicians will oppose changes they perceive as threatening their self-esteem, sense of competence, or autonomy." Does this explain the general disregard of patient and family wishes, of other practitioner's recommendations, and of denial of common sense when a patient is obviously dying? Does it come down to the preservation of one person's ego in exchange for a costly, agonizing, high-tech death as opposed to a pain-free natural occurrence?

Obviously, these issues can become very complicated and emotionally charged, and the insurance industry, with managed care leading the effort to control expenses at all costs, has decided to throw its own monkey wrench into the works - namely capitated fees. With physicians and hospitals receiving one flat fee to treat a patient's disease, a quick death translates to higher profit margins. So while we may wish to guard against the over-zealous treatment of some physicians, we now must also protect ourselves from those who are encouraged to limit treatment to maximize personal income.

Insurance companies are now going so far as to invest in our deaths when we become certifiably terminal. Viatical settlements, where a company purchases your death benefits at a 50% to 85% discount is the new wave in profiteering off of illness and suffering. The company literally buys you out, takes over your premium payments, and hopes you die soon to maximize the return on their investment. Yes, you may receive some short-term monetary relief so you may pay your inflated medical bills, but something about gambling on the date stamped on your death certificate doesn't sit well with me. The sooner you die, the sooner they can cash in your chips, leaving nothing for your previously named beneficiaries.

It's clear we need to somehow strike a balance between needlessly treating the terminally ill, and abandoning those who are salvageable. And, with the ethics of treatment being determined in a profit-driven economy these issues continue to be obscured by human vanity, ego, and greed.

Final Remarks

I challenge any politician to do something constructive for healthcare. The Democrats have failed miserably with their own plan, and now have no plan. The Republicans seem to want to privatize everything - sell it off to the highest bidder. Well, I end this book with a challenge.

I challenge those in any capacity of policy formation to do something truly constructive for patients in this country. I challenge all of the so-called leaders to open access for healthcare to all. I challenge those making our laws to open up the closed doors of institutions - make them publish their morbidity and mortality statistics, their records of malpractice, their financial statements, their investments, and their tax returns. I challenge these industry leaders to let the public know what their staffing ratios are - how many RNs do you have to take care of us? What is your ratio of administrators to patients? Is it higher than the number of RNs to patients?

I challenge any so-called nursing association to advocate for the staff nurses which are fighting for their patients. Stop playing your politically correct games to gain personal leverage while abandoning the remainder of the profession to fend for itself.

Most of all, I challenge those in power to act like morally responsible adults. This sandbox which you play in involves suffering and sacrifice - life and death.

And finally, I prescribe a dose of compassion for us all...........

*****

Bibliography

American Nurses Association. (September, 1994). Hospital Profits Soar: ANA Says RN Cutbacks Unsafe as a Way to Boost Bottom Line. The American Nurse, 30.

American Nurses Publishing. (1994). Registered Professional Nurses and Unlicensed Assistive Personnel. Washington, D.C.

Anders, G. (1994). More Members Help HMOs' Healthy Cash Flow. The Wall Street Journal, December 23, 1994.

Anders, G. (1995). Medical Boards In '94 Disciplined 12% More Doctors. The Wall Street Journal, April 6, page B7.

Anders, G. (1995). Drug Makers Help Manage Patient Care: Who Will Manage These Diseases? The Wall Street Journal, May 1995.

Associated Press. (1995). Justice Opens Two Criminal Inquires Of Tobacco Industry. Columbia Daily Tribune, July 25, page A2.

Associated Press. (1995). Organs Stolen From Living Humans In India. St. Louis Post-Dispatch, April 12, 1995, p. 25F.

Associated Press. (1995). Hospitals Asked to Refund Money. Columbia Daily Tribune, September 18, page 3B.

Baley, A. (1995). Healers' Incomes. The Kansas City Star, January 21, 1995.

Barritt, E. R. (1984). Inbreeding, Infighting, and Impotence... "Old Girls' Clubs That Have Found Their Way Into Nursing. American Journal of Nursing, 84(6), 803-804.

Bates, D. W., et al. (1995). Incidence of Adverse Drug Events and Potential Adverse Drug Events: Implications for Prevention. Journal of the American Medical Association, 274(1), 29-34.

Benton, D. A. (91986). Battered Women: Why Do They Stay? Health Care for Women International, 7(6), 403-411.

Beyers, M., Hill B. M., McCelland, M. R. & Wesley, M. L. (1992). New Wave Nursing: Back To The Basics. Nursing Clinics of North America, 27(1), 1-10.

Bickler, B. (1994). Putting Patient Focused Care Into Practice. American Operating Room Nurses Journal, 60(2), 242-245.

Bishop, J. E. (1995). AMA Urges FDA Regulation Of Tobacco. The Wall Street Journal, July 14, Page B3.

Borel, H. (1992). Powerquake! The Registered Nurse as Independent Contractor...The Mother of all Healthcare Revolutions. REVOLUTION: The Journal of Nurse Empowerment, 2(4), 25-26.

Bower, C. (1994, August 29th). Union Loses One Election at DePaul: Another Vote in Limbo. St. Louis Post-Dispatch.

Bowsher, C. A. (1991). U.S. Health Care Spending: Trends, Contributing Factors, and Proposals for Reform. Statement Before the Committee on Ways and Means, House of Representatives, Washington, D.C.

Boyd, J. W., & Himmelstein, D. U. (1995). The Tobacco Health Insurance Connection. The Lancet, July 8, Page 64.

Brett, J. L. & Tonges, M. C. (1990). Restructured Patient Care Delivery: Evaluation of the ProAct Model. Nursing Economics, 8(1), 36-44.

Bunch, D. (91992). It's All In How You Look At It: Two RTs Report on the Perceived Progress of Hospital Restructuring Projects. AARC Times, 16(8), 54-56.

Bunis, D. (1995). Rift in Nurses' Ranks Over Replacement RNs. Newsday, March 7th, p. A33-A36.

Burda, D. (1989). Union Nurses Earn More - Study. Modern Healthcare, 19(33), 4.

Burns, J. (1995). Feds Come Knocking in Search of Home-Care Fraud. Modern Healthcare, 25(23), 40- 44.

Califano, J. A. (1995). Health Care: Ministry, Not Industry. The New York Times, March 26, 1995, p. A29.

Calvin, T. (September, 1994). The Silent Epidemic: Crime in Hospitals. Good Housekeeping, 107, 258-261.

Carton, B. (1995). Bard Ex-Officials Are Found Guilty In Catheter Case. The Wall Street Journal, August 25, page B8.

Castiglia, T. C. (1992). Jealousy. Journal of Pediatric Health Care, 6(4), 212-213.

Cerne, F. (1995). Cash Kings. Hospitals and Health Networks, April 5, p. 51-54.

Chapman, J. (1993). Collegial Support Linked To Reduction Of Job Stress. Nursing Management, 24(5), 52-54.

Chipman, D. (1993). Strike! REVOLUTION - The Journal of Nurse Empowerment, 3(4), 22-25, 81-83.

Clymer, A. (1995). Medicare Cuts Create Concern. Columbia Missourian (The New York Times News Service), August 18, page 10A.

Crowley, G., Rosenburg, D., & Brant, M. (1995). The Prescription That Kills. Newsweek, July 17, page 54.

Curtin, L. (1995). Doctor Godfather. Nursing Management, 26(8), 7-8.

Emanuel, E. J.,& Steiner, D. (1995). Institutional Conflict of Interest. The New England Journal of Medicine, 332(4), 262-267.

Eubanks, P. (1990). Avoiding Unions: Supervisors are the First Line of Defense. Hospitals, 64(22), 40, 42-43.

Farris, B. J. (1993). Converting a Unit to Patient-Focused Care. Health Progress, 74(3), 22-25.

Fenner, K. M. (1991). Unionization: Boon or Bane? Journal of Nursing Administration, 21(6), 7-8.

Fralic, M. F. (1992). Creating New Practice Models and Designing New Roles: Reflections and Recommendations. Journal of Nursing Administration, 22(6), 7-8.

Gardner, J. (1995). Medicaid Plan Could Rim Medicare. Modern Healthcare, June 5, 1995, p. 34.

Gelb, B. D. (1994). Consequences of Bad Publicity: One Example. Hospital and Health Services Administration, 39(4), 435- 449.

Georges, C. & McGinley, L. (1995). Medicare Drive Toward Managed-Care System Could Turn Out To Produce A Costly Success. The Wall Street Journal, July 31, page A16.

Gordon, S. (1993). Healthcare Reform - How "The System" Works Against Nurses. REVOLUTION: The Journal of Nurse Empowerment, 3(3), 10-16, 97.

Hanrahan, T. F. (1991). Issues Related to the Use of Nurse Extenders. Journal of Nursing Administration, 21(10), 40-45.

Hayward, S. (1995). Mexican Hospital Plagued by Deaths. <u>Associated Press</u>, (date unknown/copies available).

Hilts, P. J. (1995). (AP) Tobacco Ads Seem To Appear Where Kids Are. <u>Columbia Missourian</u>, August 3, page 8A.

Hussman, M. (1995). Single-Payer System Provides Better Care. <u>The Columbia Missourian</u>, April, 1995.

Jacox, A. (1987). The OTA Report: A Policy Analysis. <u>Nursing Outlook</u>, <u>35</u>(5), 262-267.

Jenny, J. (1990). Self-Esteem: A Problem for Nurses. <u>Canadian Nurse</u>, <u>86</u>(10), 19-21.

Kelly, G. & Freundlich, N. (1992, November 2). Is There A Family Doctor In The House? <u>Business Week</u>, pp.. 124-125.

Kessler, D. A., et. al. (1994). Therapeutic Class Wars - Drug Promotion in a Competitive Marketplace. <u>The New England Journal of Medicine</u>, <u>331</u>(20), 1350- 1353.

Kimball, H. R. (1995). Credentials Misrepresentation: Another Challenge to Professionalism. <u>Annals of Internal Medicine</u>, <u>123</u>(1), 58.

Koretz, G. (1995). Look Again At Medical Bills: The Recent U.S. Dip May Not Last. <u>Business Week</u>, August 28, page 24.

Lamm, R. D. (1994). Healthcare Heresies. <u>Healthcare Forum Journal</u>, <u>37</u>(5), 45-61.

Leape, L. L. (1994). Error In Medicine. <u>Journal of The American Medical Association</u>, <u>272</u>(23), 1851-1857.

Leape, L. L., et al. (1995). Systems Analysis of Adverse Drug Events. <u>Journal of the American Medical Association</u>, <u>274</u>(1), 35-43.

Lehr, H. & Strosberg, M. (1991). Quality Improvement in Health Care: Is the Patient Still Left Out? <u>Quality Review Bulletin</u>, <u>17</u>(10), 326-329.

Manthey, M. (1988). Primary Practice Partner (A Nurse Extender System). <u>Nursing Management</u>, <u>19</u>(3), 58-59.

Manthey, M. (1989). Practice Partnerships: The Newest Concept in Care Delivery. <u>Journal of Nursing Administration</u>, <u>19</u>(2), 33-35.

Mariner, J. D. (1992). Problems With Employer Provided Insurance - The Employment Retirement Income Security Act and Health Care Reform, <u>The New</u>

England Journal of Medicine, 327(23), 1682-1685.

Marquis, B. L. & Huston, C. J. (1994). Motivation to Join or Reject Unions. Journal of Nursing Administration, 24(2), 4.

McGinley, L. (1995). GOP Overhaul of Medicare Could Be A Windfall For Insurance Firms Because of Voucher System. The Wall Street Journal, August 4, page A12.

McGinn, N. (1992). Restructuring Patient Care Delivery Systems Through Empowerment. Journal of Nursing Administration, 22(4), 21.

McLeod, B. W. (1995). The Issue of the Future - And Today. Columbia Missourian (San Francisco Examiner), August 25, page 4A.

Metzger, G. & Simpson, J. (1995). Memo: Nurses March on Washington, D.C. - Network with Directors of Nursing. The Missouri Hospital Association.

Miller, J. (1992). Use of Unlicensed Assistive Personnel in Acute Care Settings. Journal of Nursing Administration, 21(9), 29-34.

Minard, F. (1988). Competition Vs. Cooperation Among Nurses. Nursing Management, 19(3), 28-30, 32.

Moore, J. D. (1995). AMA Proposals Aim to Bolster Doc Standing. Modern Healthcare, June, 19, page 32.

Nemes, J. (1993). The Fight Against Fraud. Modern Healthcare, 23(33), 39-44.

Noah, T. & Kuntz, P. (1995). Democrats Take Aim At The Tobacco Industry, A Big Contributor To Republican Party Causes. The Wall Street Journal, July 26, Page A14.

Norris, M. K. & House M. A. (1991). Organ and Tissue Transplantation. F. A. Davis Company, Philadelphia, Pennsylvania.

Porter-O'Grady, T. (1992). Of Rabbits and Turtles: A Time of Change for Unions. Nursing Economics, 10(3), 177-182.

Porter-O'Grady, T. (1992). At Issue: Dysfunctional People In Management Roles. Aspen's Advisor for Nurse Executives, 7(9), 1, 3.

Porter-O-Grady, T. (1993). Patient-Focused Care Service Models and Nursing: Perils and Possibilities. Journal of Nursing Administration, 23(3), 7-8, 15.

Prescott, P. A. (1993). Nursing: An Important Component of Hospital Survival Under a Reformed Health Care System. Nursing Economic$, 11(4), 192- 198.

Pretzer, M. (1994). National Practitioners Data Bank -Editorial. Medical Economics, 71(18), 81- 89.

Richardson, T. (1994). Patient-Focused Care (A United Nurses of Alberta Study) Alberta, Canada: The United Nurses of Alberta Union.

Robinson, N. C. (1991). A Patient-Centered Framework for Restructuring Care. Journal of Nursing Administration, 21(9), 29-34.

Schrier, R. W. (1994). The Drug Dosing Crisis. Hospital Practice, November 15, 1994, p.11.

Schulte, F., & Bergal J. (1994). Profits From Pain. The Sun-Sentinel, December 11-15, 1994.

Sekas, G. & Hutson, W. R. (1995). Misrepresentation of Academic Accomplishments by Applicants for Gastroenterology Fellowships. Annals of Internal Medicine, 123(1), 38-59.

Schatz. T. A. (1995). Medicare Fraud: Tales From the Gypped. The Wall Street Journal, August 25, page B8.

Sheely, S. B. (1990). Mosby's Manual of Emergency Care. St. Louis.

Sherer, J. L. (1995). Managing Chaos. Hospitals and Health Networks, February 20th, 22-27.

Simpson, R. L. (1994). How Technology Can Encourage Collaborative Practice. Nursing Administrative Quarterly, 18(4), 70-83.

Smith, I. (1994). RT Roundtable: Patient-Focused Care. But Does It Really Work? RT: The Journal for Respiratory Care Practitioners, 7(3), 77-79, 80, 82.

Solovy, A. T. (1993). Champions of Change. Hospitals, 67(5), 14-19.

Staff. (1995). Workplace Briefs. The American Nurse, 27(2), 12, 15.

Staff: California Nurses Association (1994). Top Ten Myths About Hospital Restructuring and HealthCare Reform. REVOLUTION - The Journal of Nurse Empowerment, 4(3), 24-25.

Staff. (1992). Wasted Health Care Dollars. Consumer Reports, 57(7), 435-451.

Staff. (1992). Health Care Crisis: The Search for Solutions. <u>Consumer Reports,</u> <u>57</u>(9), 579-593.

Staff. (1994). INA & U. of I. Reach Agreement in O.I. Negotiations! <u>The Needle,</u> December 29th.

Staff: The American Organization of Nurse Executives (1993). When Work Redesign Prompts Unionization Activity. <u>Nursing Management,</u> <u>24</u>(9), 36-38.

Staff. (1993). Hospital Downsizing Has Special Risks. <u>Nursingworld Journal,</u> <u>19</u>(12), 1-2, 6.

Staff. (1995). <u>Rockland Journal-News,</u> Issues dating from January 5th to March 1st, 1995.

Staff. (1995). <u>The Times Herald Record,</u> Issues dating from February 25th to March 4th.

Staff. (1994). Surgeons Want Single-Payer Plan. <u>The Washington Post,</u> February 11, 1994.

Stearley, H. (1994). Gift of Life Comes With a High Price. <u>Columbia Daily Tribune,</u> January 16, 1994, p. 3D.

Stickler, K. B. (1990). Union Organizing will be Divisive and Costly. <u>Hospitals,</u> <u>64</u>(13), 68-70.

Stillwaggon, C. A. (1989). The Impact of Nurse Managed Care on the Cost of Nurse Practice and Nurse Satisfaction. <u>Journal of Nursing Administration,</u> <u>19</u>(11), 21-27.

Stout, H. (1995). Drug Firms Boosted Donations to GOP Before Vote on Bill. <u>The Wall Street Journal,</u> June 16, 1995.

Tammelleo, J. D. (ed.) (1990). Nurse Makes "Anonymous Call": Freedom of Speech. <u>The Regan Report on Nursing Law,</u> <u>31</u>(3), 1.

Tammelleo, A. D. (ed.) (1991). Supreme Court Affirms 8 Bargaining Units Per Hospital. <u>The Regan Report on Nursing Law,</u> <u>32</u>(1), 1.

Tammelleo, J. D. (ed.) (1993). Nurse Opines On Non-Natural Childbirth: Freedom of Speech. <u>The Regan Report on Nursing Law,</u> <u>34</u>(2), 1.

Tammelleo, J. D. (ed.) (1993). Nurse Refuses To "Stay Out Of It": Termination. <u>The Regan Report on Nursing Law,</u> <u>34</u>(2), 4.

Tammelleo, J. D. (ed.) (1994). "Patient Endangerment" Remark -Termination: Free Speech. <u>The Regan Report on Nursing Law,</u> <u>35</u>(6), 1.

The Regan Report on Nursing Law, 35(2), 1.

Tammelleo, J. D. (ed.) (1994). Supreme Court Rules NLRB Erred Re "Supervisory Nurses". The Regan Report on Nursing Law, 35(2), 1.

Taunton, R. L., et al. (1994). Patient Outcomes: Are They Linked to Registered Nurse Absenteeism, Separation, or Workload? Journal of Nursing Administration, 24(4S), 48-55.

Townsend, M. B. (1993). Patient-focused Care; Is It For Your Hospital? Nursing Management, 24(9), 74-80.

Trimpley, M. L. (1989). Self-Esteem and Anxiety: Key Issues in an Abused Women's Support Group. Issues in Mental Health Nursing, 10(3), 297-308.

Urlich, Y. C. (1991). Women's Reasons for Leaving Abusive Spouses. Health Care for Women International, 12(4), 465-473.

U. S. Department of Health and Human Services (1993). Questions and Answers About Organ Transplantation. U. S. Government Printing Office, 1993-0-305-247.

United States General Accounting Office (1992). Medicare Claims. Report # GAO/HR- 93-6.

University of Missouri Curators. (1995). The University of Missouri System: Fiscal 1995 Operating Budget.

Wachter, R. M. (1995). Rationing Health Care: Preparing for a New Era. Southern Medical Journal, 88(1), 25-32.

Walter, R. (1994). Under the Influence: The Myth of Professional Codependency. REVOLUTION: The Journal of Nurse Empowerment, 4(2), 69-71.

Wang, P. (1992, March). Nine Out Of Ten Hospital Bills Are Wrong: Here's How to Spot Mistakes And Get A Refund. Money, pp. 138-142.

Weber, D. O. (1993). Well? Healthcare Forum Journal, 36(6), 41-55.

Weber, D. O. (1994). Health Herstory. Healthcare Forum Journal, 37(1), 41-47.

Weissenstein E. (1995). HCFA Proposes 20% Rise In Capital Rates. Modern Healthcare, June 5, 1995, p. 4.

Welt, S. R. (1987). The Physchodynamics of Envy: Part 4. Archives of Psychiatric Nursing, 1(5), 322-333.

Williams, W. E. (1995). Who Gets Organs Should Be Decided on the Market. The

Williams, W. E. (1995). Who Gets Organs Should Be Decided on the Market. <u>The Columbia Daily Tribune</u>, June 25, 1995, p. 7A.

Wilson, C. N., Hamilton, C. L., & Murphy, E. (1990). Union Dynamics in Nursing. <u>Journal of Nursing Administration</u>, <u>20</u>(2), 35-39.

Winslow, R. (1995). Drug-Industry Sales Pitches to Doctors are Inaccurate 11% of Times, Study Says. <u>The Wall Street Journal</u>, (date unknown/copies available).

Woititz, J. G. (1989). <u>The Self- Sabotage Syndrome: Adult Children in the Workplace</u>. Deerfield Beach, Florida: Health Communications.

Bio-Note

Harold Stearley, R.N., B.S.N., A.S.B., CCRN, has held various clinical and supervisory positions over his twenty-two year career, and has helped develop innovative programs for several hospitals. He is a member of Sigma Theta Tau, and was named in "Who's Who in Nursing" and Who's Who in America." His freelance writing appears regularly in the local press in Missouri, and his articles have been featured in *Nursing, Nursing Administrative Quarterly, Nursing Economics, Journal of Nursing Jocularity, The Missouri Nurse*, and *REVOLUTION - The Journal of Nurse Empowerment*. He holds positions on the Editorial Board of The Missouri Nurse, and on the Staff Nurse Editorial Advisory Board for The American Nurse.

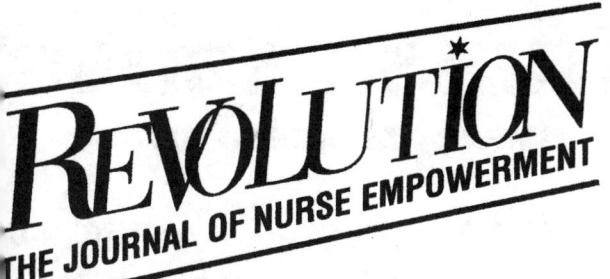

$24.95 / year
Quarterly Journal
$44.95 / year
Hospital / Institution

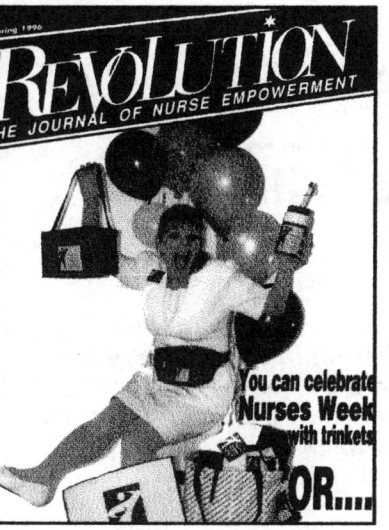

Hospital Practices That Erode Nursing Power
Manipulation and deceit keep hospitals in power and nurses disenfranchised.

Are Nurses Destined To Be A Dying Breed?
What the government isn't telling nurses about AIDS is what the hospital isn't protecting them against.

Making History: The RN/CEO
How one nurse's "Good Idea" turned into a 15 million dollar business.

Legislative Update
We will keep you updated on the bills and legislation in Washington D.C., and their impact on the nursing profession.

Toward A Feminist Model For The Political Empowerment Of Nurses
A look at some old questions about the male-dominated system of power and the inequality between nursing administration and staff nurses.

The Nurse Who Doesn't Exist: Omission and Neglect of Nurses In The Media
Why are nurses so ignored by the media? An expert offers some shocking statistics, piercing insights and suggested solutions.

If you feel the nursing profession is worth fighting for
JOIN THE REVOLUTION

An award winning quarterly journal, over 100 full color pages, that focuses on the academic, clinical, personal and political issues that effect registered nurses.

WE TELL IT LIKE IT IS! AND WE'RE CHANGING THE "SYSTEM"!

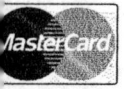
Call 1-800-331-6534
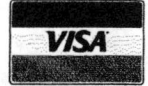

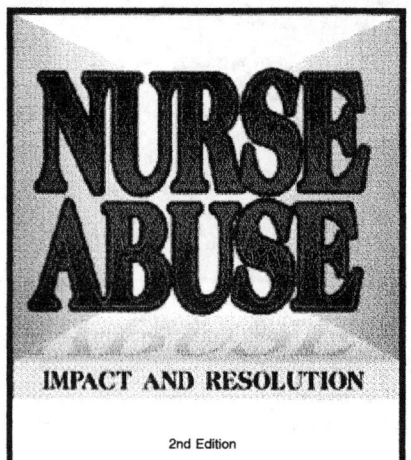

NURSE ABUSE
IMPACT AND RESOLUTION

This 300+ page book focuses on the frustrations, problems and barriers confronting nurses, as well as offering solutions

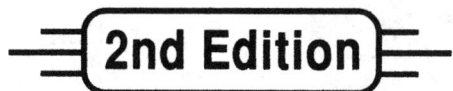

"NURSE ABUSE: IMPACT AND RESOLUTION" *is a compilation of essays that are the authors' personal reflection of a profession in crisis. It represents a combined effort of staff nurses, nurse administrators, professors of nursing and nurse researchers who focused on some of the special issues, problems and barriers confronting nurses, as well as offering possible solutions.*

Editors:

Laura Gasparis Vonfrolio, RN, PhD, CEN, CCRN
Joan Swirsky, RN, MS, CS
Harold Stearley, RN
With Contributing Authors

$24.95 plus $3.00 Shipping and Handling

To order **NURSE ABUSE** please make checks or money orders payable to:
Power Publications
56 McArthur Avenue, Staten Island, NY 10312

Name: _____ Telephone No: _____

Address: _____

City: _____ State: _____ Zip: _____

Payment must accompany this order form.

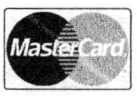

Call 1-800-331-6534

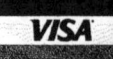